MW01065501

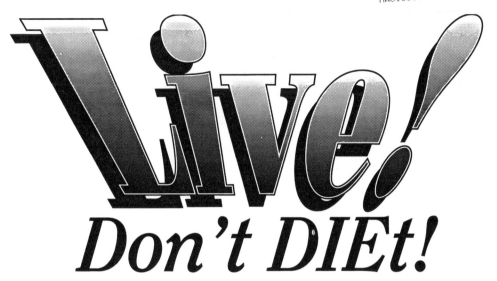

Don't DIEt!

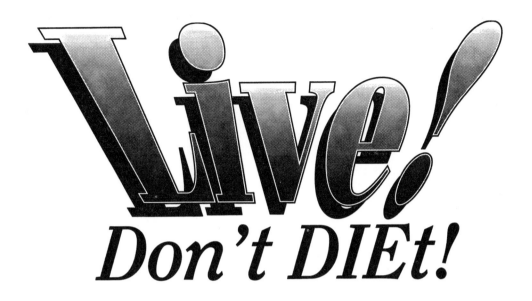

Live! Don't DIEt!

The Low-fat Cookbook
That Can Change
Your Life!

Vicki Park

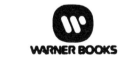

WARNER BOOKS

A Time Warner Company

Neither this diet/nor any other diet program should be followed without first consulting a health care professional. If you have any special conditions requiring attention, you should consult with your health care professional regularly regarding possible modification of the program contained in this book.

Warner Books Edition
Copyright © 1995 by PepperTree Press
All rights reserved.

This Warner Books edition is published by arrangement with Peppertree Press, P.O. Box 232, Pleasant Grove, AL 35127

Warner Books, Inc., 1271 Avenue of the Americas, New York, NY 10020

A Time Warner Company

Printed in the United States of America
First Warner Books Printing: February 1996
10 9 8 7 6 5 4

Library of Congress Cataloging-in-Publication Data
Park, Vicki.
    Live, don't diet! : the low-fat cookbook that can change your
life! / Vicki Park.
       p. cm.
    Originally published : Pleasant Grove, Ala. : PepperTree Press, 1995.
    Includes index.
    ISBN 0-446-67229-7 (pbk.)
    1. Low-fat diet—Recipes.   2. Reducing diets. I. Title.
[RM237.7.P35   1996]
641.5'638—dc20
                                      95-35775
                                          CIP

Cover photography by Spider Martin
Book design by Lori Leath-Smith

I dedicate this book to my family who has loved me and supported me through thick (and at 315 pounds, I do mean thick!) and thin, and to the memory of my Dad, Virgil Whatley.

A Special Thank You

My special thanks and deepest gratitude to my husband, Ken; my daughter, Ashley; my mom, Lorene Whatley; my in-laws, Elmer and Odell Park; my aunt, Lou Renfroe; my cousin, Jan Moore; and to Helen Davis, Steve Parker, Jim Lunsford, Lori Leath-Smith, Bill Stokes, Don Pippen, Spider Martin, Michael Dulin, Randy West, Cherie Kosak, Tom Moore, and Ann Isaac. Your hard work, guidance, faith, and encouragement are appreciated more than words can say.

Table of Contents

Preface

Isn't it an amazing coincidence that the word diet starts with die and has a cross at the end? It certainly is appropriate. If you diet, you feel as though you are starving to death. If you don't diet, your excess weight may eventually kill you. Even if you are not overweight, the dismal reports on the health dangers of many favorite foods make you wonder if you are killing yourself if you don't change to a healthier diet. It is an awful dilemma. I should know. I spent most of my life dieting, yet I ended up weighing 315 pounds. Conventional diets weren't working for me and my favorite non-diet foods were probably killing me. I was in a constant state of guilt, fear and frustration.

That was all before I learned about weight loss the low-fat way. As a last resort, I decided to give it a try. I figured that even if I didn't lose an ounce, I would at least be eating right. I never in my wildest dreams imagined that I would end up losing more than 165 pounds!

Many people ask me to tell them how I lost weight. I am the first to admit that I am no expert. I am not a doctor nor am I a nutritionist. I am just an average person. My life may be a lot like yours. I'm a working mother, with too much to do and too little time to spend hours in the kitchen. I love to eat. I have no willpower. I hate to exercise. Yet I lost 165 pounds by learning to prepare tasty, simple low-fat dishes that satisfied me and my family. No, I am not an expert, nor do I have miraculous solutions. I cannot guarantee that everyone will lose. However, I can share the benefit of my personal experience in losing 165 pounds through low-fat eating. That is one thing even most experts can't do. In addition I can offer you the low-fat recipes, cooking techniques and low-fat eating tips that I used to lose.

Low-fat eating literally saved my life. It is so easy and fulfilling to me that I cannot imagine ever going back to my old eating habits. Whether you want to lose weight, or just want to eat healthier, I hope you will find something in this book to help you. I also hope that you will find low-fat living as easy and as rewarding as I have.

How I Lost Weight the Low-fat Way

Why Try?

How I Lost More Than 165 Pounds

What The Low-fat Lifestyle Is Not

Some Additional Tips About Low-fat Weight Loss

WHY TRY?

In this day and time, it has become accepted wisdom that if you are satisfied with being overweight and are in reasonably good health, you should just forget about trying to lose. Perhaps that might work for some people, but it never worked for me. While I had tried just about every diet around and had finally given up trying, I was always nagged by the feeling that I should try again. However, I would never do anything about it. I just ate and ate and felt guilty. I worried about developing weight related health problems such as diabetes or heart trouble. I also worried about being an embarrassment to my family, although they are so sweet, they would never admit that I was. Unfortunately, worrying was all I did. It didn't motivate me to try to take the weight off.

In order to succeed at weight loss, most of us have to have a very personal reason. We all know that extra weight can cause health problems. In addition, society often discriminates against overweight people. However, that hasn't kept 50 million of us from holding on to those extra pounds. It isn't enough that someone else wants us to lose. We have to want to do it for ourselves. We have to find an intensely motivating personal reason to lose.

What pushed me into trying again? I simply realized that food had become the only exciting thing in my life. Once I came to this conclusion, I knew that I had to do something about it. I was missing out on so much! I was always tired and unhappy, because I was so fat. I didn't go a lot of places, such as the beach, because I was so fat. I avoided many social situations, because I was so fat. All I enjoyed and looked forward to was my next meal. I had allowed food to take center stage in my life.

Today, I love to get out and go. I have energy. I have rediscovered the excitement life can offer. I still love to eat, but now I control my food—it doesn't control me!

Find your own personal reason to want to lose. Keep that reason front and center in your mind at all times. It will be a motivating force that will lead you to weight loss success.

How I Lost More Than 165 Pounds

Who among us has not wished for a magic diet that would allow us to lose weight, while filling up on delicious, hearty food? The wishing is over. It is here now. However, it is not a diet in the conventional sense. It is simply a change to healthier eating habits. It has been referred to as a low-fat lifestyle. If you follow a low-fat lifestyle, you simply get rid of most of the fat in your food. You forget about deprivation, and eating "rabbit" food. You concentrate on filling up on delicious and hearty foods like vegetables, potatoes, pasta and bread in quantities that have always been taboo on conventional diets.

A friend once told me that when she joined a popular diet program, she was given a list of foods she could eat each day. "What can I do if I am still hungry when this is gone?" she asked the counselor. "Go to bed!" the counselor replied. That says it all. That is why I have never been able to stay on a conventional diet. Subconsciously, I can't handle any limit being placed on how much I can eat. Once the limit is imposed, I begin to feel deprived. I stay hungry and crave forbidden foods. That is why I could seldom stay on a conventional diet more than a few days.

The low-fat lifestyle changed all that for me. I am free to eat until I am full. I am able to handle cravings because I can fit almost any temptation into my daily fat allowance, or I can create low-fat variations, using the wonderful low-fat and fat-free substitutes now on the market.

Simply put, I lost the weight because I stopped eating fatty foods. Losing weight by reducing fat intake is certainly not a new concept. It has been widely studied and recommended by medical experts. Many feel that it is the best hope for successful long-term weight loss. There are a number of good books by physicians and nutritionists available on low-fat weight loss. While they all advise cutting fat intake to lose weight, they vary somewhat in their approach.

If you are thinking about reducing your fat intake in order to lose weight, go to the public library or bookstore and check out some books on the subject. Read them and come to your own conclusions about which plan is best for you. Of course, no one should ever make a change in eating habits without consulting a physician. Be sure to talk to your own physician before reducing your fat intake. Ask how many fat grams you should allow yourself. Also, ask if you need a vitamin supplement. Since all individuals are different, your physician's advice and consent is essential. I personally chose to limit my fat intake to a minimum of 25 grams and a maximum of 35 grams per day. Some doctors advise the elimination of meat in a low-fat eating plan, others do not. I chose not to exclude any foods. If I don't eat something, it is just because I don't want it, not that I can't have it. I feel that this approach is best for me because it is so similar to my old eating habits. I only had to modify my old, favorite recipes with low-fat ingredients. This is also why I feel confident that I won't go back to my old eating habits. As I said before, this is not really a diet. It is simply a change to healthier eating habits. It is amazing that something so easy could have such a profound effect on my life.

WHAT THE LOW–FAT LIFESTYLE IS NOT

"Please try just a little of this cake, it's low-fat," my well meaning friend said. "I'm watching my fat intake so I made it with only one stick of butter instead of two." Her misconception is not uncommon. Many people think they can lose weight by cutting out just a little fat. A low-fat lifestyle is not just dropping a few fat grams here and there. It is a commitment to low-fat eating as a way of life. It is also not a roller coaster ride of low-fat eating one day and high-fat the next. The media likes to point out that the 1990's are a time of contradictions food-wise. People will eat a prudent, healthy meal, then stuff themselves with an extravagant, fat-laden dessert. You can't lose much weight this way. Remember, this is a lifestyle, not one day on and one day off.

The low-fat lifestyle is also not a license to gorge. A friend of mine could not understand why she wasn't losing weight when she began watching her fat intake. It didn't take much detective work to discover why. She would habitually sit down and eat a whole bag of fat-free cookies while watching television at night. You need to stay away from too many sugary treats, even if they are low-fat. The low-fat lifestyle can allow you to lose weight because you fill up and stay full by eating a lot of complex carbohydrates and protein. Occasionally you might pig out on low-fat goodies, but, in general, moderation is the key to consistent weight loss. Eat only until you are comfortably full, not until you are ready to pop!

The low-fat lifestyle is not a quick fix. I lost at an average rate of about 10 pounds per month. It was not a constant 10 pounds. Some months I lost less and some months I lost more. You don't want to lose too fast. The more slowly it comes off, the more likely it will stay off. Don't get impatient!

When I first decided to see if low-fat eating would help me lose weight, I told myself I would just eat all I wanted, while staying within my allotted fat grams. I told myself that if I lost weight, it would be great, but if I didn't, I would at least be eating foods that were good for me. After all, every day new reports come out about the health benefits of a low-fat lifestyle. I didn't put myself under any pressure to lose. I just ate low-fat foods and the weight and inches started to come off. Everyone is different. There are no guarantees that everyone will lose, but it worked for me and may work for you. Don't put pressure on yourself. Just tell yourself that by eating plenty of delicious, low-fat foods, you will almost certainly be treating your body better. The weight you may lose will just be a wonderful dividend.

SOME ADDITIONAL TIPS ABOUT LOW-FAT WEIGHT LOSS

Since I have lived with a low-fat lifestyle for more than two years, I have learned quite a lot about what to expect in terms of weight loss. In addition to the personal experiences that I have already shared with you, I can add a few more things that I have learned.

1. Weigh seldom, if ever. It is really best to get rid of your bathroom scale. It is a seductive enemy. It lures you to weigh, then dashes your hopes if you haven't lost. Weight is not a stable thing. You may actually be losing, but due to normal fluid retention, may appear to be gaining. If you don't weigh, you won't worry. You won't be tempted to quit. I am sorry to say that I came to this realization only after I had lost the weight. I didn't know any better, so I did weigh. If I had not lost, I would get depressed. That is why I know it isn't a good thing to weigh. It is better to measure yourself around the chest, waist, hips, thighs and upper arms. Then measure again from time to time. Even when you are not losing pounds, you may be losing body fat. As strange as that sounds, that happened to me. You may even want to buy a caliper to measure body fat. That is what doctors use. You can also tell when

you are losing by the fit of your clothes.

2. I found that weight loss is a little different with a low-fat lifestyle than with a conventional diet. I lost in spurts. That is another reason it is important not to weigh. I would think I was never going to lose another ounce, then suddenly 10 pounds would drop off. I averaged losing 10 pounds per month. However, even when my weight loss slowed down, I would continue to lose inches. That is why it is important to measure periodically.

3. Be sure to eat plenty of high-fiber foods, including dry beans, whole grains, fruits and vegetables. They not only keep you full, they help prevent irregularity. Some people may experience bloating when they begin eating a lot of fiber. This can usually be avoided by increasing fiber intake gradually.

4. If you are still hungry at the end of a meal, wait a few minutes before eating more. Sometimes even a short break can make you realize that you are really full after all.

5. Remember this old saying, if you are tempted to stray from your low-fat lifestyle: **Nothing tastes as good as being thinner feels!**

The Voice of Experience

Useful Tips I've Learned About Low-fat Living

SUBSTITUTE! SUBSTITUTE! SUBSTITUTE!

Several years ago, I bought some fat-free cheese. After one bite, I threw it away. But then, several years ago, I weighed 315 pounds. Today I love fat-free cheese. I also weigh more than 165 pounds less than I did then. It's a trade off; fatty foods-fatty body, low-fat foods-low-fat body.

I recently read a cooking magazine in which there was a letter from an irate reader to the editor berating the magazine staff for saying that their low-fat version of tortilla chips was better tasting than fried, commercially prepared chips. There is a quality about fat that makes foods without it seem as though something is missing. Just think about it. If our foods do not naturally contain fat, we have to pile on the oil or butter, even though it provides little, if any additional taste.

Food experts call that something that fat adds to foods, "mouth-feel." This refers to the smooth, oily richness that fat imparts. It gives foods a full-bodied, satisfying taste that makes people naturally prefer them over low-fat foods. In a taste test, head to head, a low-fat or fat-free version of a food will probably seldom win over the original. The trick is to never let yourself make the comparison. It is the best thing you can possibly do for yourself if you want to be successful in following a low-fat lifestyle.

These are words to live by: I WILL NOT LET MYSELF COMPARE THE TASTE OF MY LOW-FAT FOODS TO THEIR HIGH-FAT COUNTERPARTS. I WILL SIMPLY ENJOY THEM, WITHOUT MAKING ANY COMPARISON. This statement is engraved on my brain. Engrave it on yours, too. It will allow you to prepare delicious, satisfying versions of your old favorites without missing the originals. You will also enjoy coming up with new ways to use substitutes in your cooking. Trips to the grocery store become an adventure. It is fun to see the new low-fat products that come out almost weekly. I especially enjoy finding new fat-free or reduced-fat dairy products. Fat-free cream cheese, sour cream, cottage cheese, and hard cheese have been mainstays in my low-fat cooking, and I anxiously await new dairy substitutes as they become available.

With my low-fat lifestyle, I am not tempted to stray back to my old eating habits because I know that I can either fit a serving of the original into my fat gram allowance, or better yet, create a reasonable facsimile of any dish that I might normally crave with low-fat substitutes. That knowledge is very liberating. On every diet that I tried before, I feared cravings. I knew that I would end up giving in to them and my diet would be history. I no longer have to fear them. They have lost their power over me. Want a hot fudge sundae? Fat-free fudge sauce and fat-free frozen yogurt with light whipped topping are so good no one would ever guess they are not the high-fat version. Crave a cheese-burger? No problem. A lower-fat version is not only possible, but delicious.

You may not believe it now, but in time you will probably come to prefer the low-fat versions of your favorites, just as the magazine staff did. You will find that you do not like the oily, greasy taste that the higher-fat originals leave in your mouth. You will become very sensitive to the unpleasant, slick sensation that fat imparts. Just think, would you eat a big spoonful of grease? Of course not. Yet when you eat a food that contains fat, you are coating your mouth with the same oily residue. This makes food taste good? I think not!!

IT'S WHAT'S UP FRONT THAT COUNTS

Have you noticed that when someone really wants you to see something, they stick it in front of you to get your attention? The same should be true with food. Often the most interesting ingredients in a dish get lost when they are mixed in with everything else. When I want to blow some of my fat grams on a teaspoon of nuts, a bit of real mayonnaise, or another special ingredient, I place it in the spotlight by putting it on top of my serving. Just a taste can seem like a lot.

An ingredient doesn't have to be high-fat to deserve to be front and center. Don't serve vegetables "topless" unless you just like them that way. Perk them up by adding a little something extra. A sprinkle of crunchy, minced dried onion, a bit of low-fat canned gravy, or a little catsup can do wonders for a plain, cooked vegetable. Even ultra-low-fat margarine can seem lavish when spread on top. It's fun to use your imagination to think up new toppings. The possibilities are endless.

How Important Is Exercise?

I am not proud to admit that I hate to exercise. I have always hated to exercise. After all, I didn't come to weigh 315 pounds by being a fitness buff. I doubt that I will ever grow to like it, but I have come to recognize that it is an important part of weight management.

I lost more than 100 pounds through low-fat eating before I ever did any exercise. I say that mainly to let you know that it is often possible to lose weight this way even if you are not physically able to exercise, or if you do not feel that you are up to beginning both a new way of eating and a fitness regimen at the same time. Weight loss is likely to be faster with exercise. Quite frankly, I probably would have never begun my low-fat lifestyle if exercise was required for it to work. I simply changed my eating habits, not my exercise habits, which were nonexistent. However, when I had lost just over 100 pounds, I hit a lengthy plateau. My weight didn't budge for several months. Since adjustments in food intake and/or exercise have always been considered classic ways to get off a weight loss plateau, I decided that exercise might be the jump start I needed to begin losing again.

I decided to give aerobic exercise a try. Experts feel that aerobic exercise for 20 minutes to one hour, three times a week or more, increases the metabolic rate and thus the rate at which our bodies burn fat. Walking, bicycling and swimming are all great aerobic exercises, but I felt I would do better with an exercise program that provided a lot of variety. I found a great exercise video that consists of several segments of simple movements. Each segment lasts about 20 minutes. I do one segment every other day. I probably should do more, but I figure that I am doing good to make myself exercise at all. The aerobics did the trick. I got off the plateau and went on to lose over 65 more pounds. I plan to continue this simple exercise program.

I also try to get "non-exercise" exercise. I park my car as far from the mall as possible. I get up from my desk and move around more at work. I push my cart at a brisk pace down the uncrowded aisles in the discount store, instead of strolling at a leisurely pace. I even sprint up the stairs several times a day.

You will have to make your own decision about exercise. You should definitely consult your doctor before embarking on any exercise program, as well as any change in eating habits. Exercise is an important part of good health. It helps you gain energy and can help you lose weight faster. There are so many kinds that you should be able to find one, or more, that is right for you. I really regret that I did not start exercising sooner. Most experts agree that exercise is the true key to permanent weight loss.

WHAT ABOUT THE REST OF THE FAMILY?

Not long after we married, my husband Ken developed a major weight problem—me. In order to impress my new husband, I prepared rich, tempting dishes for every meal. I also kept the pantry stocked with his favorite goodies. While my weight zoomed immediately, he was more fortunate. Because he was more active, he was able to maintain a reasonable weight while eating a lot of fattening foods. As the years passed, however, his luck changed. By the time we celebrated our 20th wedding anniversary, he weighed almost 250 pounds, while I weighed more than 300. Needless to say, neither of us had ever had much luck with our attempts at conventional dieting.

When I made the decision to serve only low-fat meals, Ken supported me all the way. While he doesn't count fat grams, he did begin to watch his fat intake. He eats only my low-fat cooking at home, and tries to select lower-fat dishes in restaurants. As a result he now weighs 175 pounds. His doctor recently removed him from the blood pressure medication that he has taken for years.

Ken is often amazed that the dishes I prepare are low in fat. During a meal, he will sometimes look at me skeptically and say, "Are you sure we can have this?" Like myself, he doesn't really miss our old high-fat eating habits.

Our daughter, Ashley, grew up with an aversion to fresh vegetables, fruits and other nutritious foods. Despite my best efforts, she is a picky eater with a passion for fast food. She is now away at college, and is delighted that she is finally free to eat pizza three times a day. However, she does admit that some of the low-fat dishes at home were not bad at all.

Many experts feel that for the average person, no more than 30% of the calories consumed daily should come from fat. Therefore other family members should benefit from low-fat meals. Ask your physician how many fat grams each member of your household needs daily.

It may vary somewhat according to sex, age and physical condition. Of course, it also can depend upon whether an individual wants to lose weight or just wants to eat healthier. In general, the same low-fat meals should work for everyone, with only minor modifications necessary to fulfill the dietary requirements of those whose fat intake needs to be a bit higher.

ARE YOU LETTING FAT ROB YOUR LIFE OF ROMANCE?

It has been said that a day without wine is like a day without sunshine. The same could be said of romance. Even in this cynical day and time, romance is an important part of life. People are hungry for it. Witness the popularity of romantic books, movies, and television shows. We can't seem to get enough of them. We seek romance vicariously, through the lives of fictional characters, often because there is not enough of it in our real lives. Romance, even when experienced through the lives of others, adds a certain zest to life. When we have our own romance, it can really add excitement. It doesn't have to be a blazing, torrid love affair. It can be as simple as a little pleasant flirting with the one we love.

It is unfortunate that the amount of romance in real life generally decreases as the amount of body fat increases. Of course, we all know that romantic attraction should be based on the inner beauty of a person, not the exterior. However, that's not reality. Right or wrong, romantic attraction is usually based on appearance. If you don't believe it, ask yourself why sexy, thin actors always play the romantic leads in movies, while overweight actors end up in the funny, but loveless best friend roles. We may feel deep spiritual love for our beloved, but if he lets himself get fat, our romantic interest in him can fade.

One rainy afternoon, I picked up a deliciously romantic novel that was enthralling. I couldn't put it down. As I finished the final page, I wondered if real life couldn't be as romantic if I worked at making it that way. Since I had let myself get up to 315 pounds, I obviously, hadn't worked at it in a long time. Romance was one of the things my life was missing because I had let fat gain control. As Ken and I both lost weight through our low-fat lifestyles, the romance did come back. It is wonderful.

Perhaps you have also let fat rob your life of romance. You may not even think that it is important in your life. Maybe it's not. But give it a chance. If the spark of romance in your soul has gone out, read a romantic book, listen to seductive music, or fall under the spell of a movie love story. One of these may relight that spark. It may motivate you to want to lose weight and perhaps bring romance back to your personal life. While losing weight isn't guaranteed to do this, it certainly won't hurt the chances of it happening. After all, who could resist the new, thinner you?

IMPROVE WHILE YOU LOSE

As you lose, you often begin to think about making other improvements in your appearance. I developed an image of how I wanted to look. I kept that image in mind every day. It helped me stay on track with my weight loss plan. I decided to make major changes in how I dressed. I had worn so many pastel prints while fat that I decided to wear more sophisticated solid color suits and dresses. I learned that good, striking jewelry will make even the plainest outfit look great, so I also began to purchase pieces that were unique. I previously bought make-up at the discount store. I decided to visit a professional and learn how to properly use the right makeup. I had never taken the least bit of care of my complexion, just leaving my face to fate, soap, and water. I visited the dermatologist and got a prescription for Retin-A, which has evened out my complexion. I also learned that daily use of sunscreen can help prevent some wrinkles.

I am no beauty now, but I do feel that the changes I made have vastly improved my appearance, as well as my self esteem. Most women would die if they heard that their husband had been seen with another woman. I was thrilled, because the other woman my husband was seen with was me! A friend gleefully related to me that a mutual acquaintance who had not seen me in a long time reported to her that my husband and I were apparently no longer together. He had been seen from a distance on several occasions with a much slimmer, more attractive woman! What a compliment!

You may find making some style and appearance changes as rewarding as I did. They can really perk up your life.

DINING OUT

I have seen books on low-fat living that devoted long, wordy chapters to dining out. Frankly, I don't have the patience to wade through all that. It is just not necessary.

Since I do not like to take my lunch to work, I have dined out almost every weekday since I began following a low-fat lifestyle. I carry a small fat gram counter in my purse. If the restaurant is one of a national chain, I can often look up the fat content of their dishes in the book.

Many full service and fast food restaurants now offer low-fat selections. If you are dining in a full service restaurant, you may also simply confide in your servers that you are watching your fat intake. They can be most helpful in making suggestions. Usually broiled entrées, such as chicken or fish, can easily be prepared without oil or butter. Other entrées may also be modified to your requirements. Order baked potatoes or vegetables plain and add catsup or lemon juice. Salads can be eaten with fat-free dressing or, if not available, with regular dressing on the side. Dip your fork into the dressing, then the greens. You get a taste of the dressing without too much fat.

I usually eat at fast food restaurants several days a week. Their grilled chicken sandwiches (without mayo), ultra-lean burgers or turkey sandwiches, along with a side salad with fat-free dressing, make a fine meal. Many of their meal-size salads are also quite low in fat.

Fat-free salad dressings are widely available in grocery stores in individual packets. I carry a supply of my favorites, as well as a shaker of fat-free butter-flavored granules, sour cream-flavored granules, and Cheddar cheese-flavored granules in a zipper top plastic bag in my car. When dining out, I can drop any or all of them into my purse and use them discreetly in the restaurant.

Tips For Cooking The Low-fat Way

REDUCING THE FAT IN YOUR RECIPES

It is really easy to lower the fat in your own favorite recipes. These are a few of the ingredients that will help you.

Original Ingredient:	Low-Fat Alternative:
Swiss or Cheddar cheese	Fat-free Swiss or Cheddar
Butter or Margarine	Ultra-light or fat-free margarine
	Butter-flavored granules
	Butter-flavored cooking spray
Eggs	Fat-free egg substitute
	Egg whites
Canned cream soup	99% fat-free canned cream soup
1 cup whole or low-fat milk	1 cup skim milk
1 cup cream or half and half	1 cup evaporated skim milk
Sour cream	Fat-free sour cream
Cream cheese	Fat-free cream cheese
Oil	No-stick cooking spray
	Applesauce (in baked goods)
	Baby food prunes (in baked goods)
Salad dressing	Fat-free salad dressing
Mayonnaise	Fat-free mayonnaise
	Fat-free salad dressing
Wieners	97% fat-free wieners
Baked ham	98% fat-free precooked ham
Ground beef	Ground top round

A Short Guide To Fat Grams

When I decided to limit my fat intake, I went to the bookstore and invested in several copies of a good fat gram guide. There are a number on the market. Most list the fat grams in thousands of foods. I keep one at home, one in the car, one at the office, and a very small one in my purse. Even after more than two years of low-fat eating, I still consult them when I need to determine the amount of fat grams in an unfamiliar food.

Counting fat grams is very easy. Just remember: plain vegetables and plain fruits (except avocado) have practically no fat. The following is a very short list of the fat grams in some other common foods. This is merely a sample. Buy at least one fat gram guide to use as a reference. You will be surprised to learn that some of your favorite foods are probably lower in fat than you think.

Breakfast Foods:

Bacon, fried	1 slice	3.1 grams
Bagel	1 whole	1.4 grams
Cornflakes	1 cup	.1 gram
Eggs	1 whole	5.0 grams

Dairy Products:

Buttermilk	1 cup	4.0 grams
Cheese, hard	1 oz.	4.9-9.4 grams
Milk, 1%	1 cup	2.6 grams
Milk, skim	1 cup	1.0 gram
Milk, whole	1 cup	8.2 grams
Sour cream	1 tablespoon	3.0 grams

Meats (trimmed of all fat):

Beef, eye of round	3 oz.	6.5 grams
Beef, ground	3 oz.	19.2 grams
Ham, extra-lean	3 oz.	4.1 grams
Lamb chop	3 oz.	32.0 grams
Pork tenderloin	3 oz.	4.1 grams

Poultry (skinless):

Chicken breast	4 oz.	5.1 grams
Turkey breast	4 oz.	1.0 grams

USING SUGAR AND SUGAR SUBSTITUTES

I have very little willpower, and when there is a dessert in the house, one piece is never enough for me. If you fill up on healthy grains, beans, vegetables and fruits, you won't really want or miss sugary desserts. When I do prepare a recipe that calls for sugar, I usually replace all or part of the sugar with sugar substitutes. You may prefer not to use them, but while I don't count calories I like to cut calories out of my recipes whenever and however possible. My recipes call for the use of saccharin-based granulated-style substitute, which replaces the sugar measure for measure. Aspartame-based substitutes are great in foods that don't require lengthy heating, but tend to lose their sweetness when used in foods that are cooked. Therefore it is best to use saccharin-based substitutes in cooked dishes. If you choose to use sugar substitutes, try these equivalents in your cooking:

Bulk granulated-style saccharin-based substitute: Measure the same as sugar.

Saccharin-based packets: ¼ cup = 3 packets, ⅓ cup = 4 packets ½ cup = 6 packets, 1 cup = 12 packets.

Bulk granulated-style aspartame-based substitute: Measure the same as sugar.

Aspartame-based packets: ¼ cup = 6 packets, ⅓ cup = 8 packets, ½ cup = 12 packets, ⅔ cup = 16 packets, 1 cup = 24 packets.

WHAT ABOUT SODIUM?

As a busy person who is not fond of spending a lot of time in the kitchen, I depend heavily on convenience foods and canned goods while preparing the meals for my low-fat lifestyle. Unfortunately, many such foods are quite high in sodium. In order to limit my family's sodium intake, I take the following steps:

1. I seldom add salt to any food. Most dishes are sufficiently salty from ingredients used in their preparation.

2. I buy only light salt. While it still has sodium, it has less than regular salt.

3. I buy a variety of the herb/spice salt replacement products that add interesting tastes to food in order to eliminate the need for salt. They come in many blends, such as onion/herb, garlic/herb and lemon/herb.

4. I drain and rinse canned vegetables. They are often high in sodium and rinsing can eliminate some of it.

5. I buy low-sodium products whenever possible. Just as new low-fat products come out almost daily, low-sodium varieties of our favorite foods are also becoming widely available. Low-sodium bouillon cubes, soy sauce, catsup, processed meats and canned goods are just a few of the products you can now find.

6. If I use a high-sodium processed meat in a recipe, I try to limit the amount used to the bare minimum.

Cooking With Ground Beef

The average ground beef sold in grocery stores can contain a lot of fat, so it has no place in a low-fat lifestyle. However, you don't have to throw out all of your old recipes that contain ground beef. There are low-fat alternatives.

One alternative is to use ground turkey instead of ground beef. If you choose to do this, make sure the ground turkey is 100 percent pure ground breast meat. The ground turkey sold in stores often contains fat or even skin. You may need to have the butcher grind turkey breast for you.

I prefer ground beef, so I buy several pounds of top round and have it trimmed of all fat and ground by the butcher. I brown it in my dutch oven, pat it with paper towels to absorb any grease, then rinse it under hot running water to remove any additional grease. The meat is so lean to start with that I have never had any problems with grease in my drain, but if you have a particularly sensitive plumbing system, you may want to skip the rinsing step. Finally, I place the meat on paper towels and pat dry. I then divide it into 6-ounce portions and freeze. When I make any casserole or sauce that calls for ground beef, I just use a 6-ounce portion of my frozen cooked ground round. Just a little does as well as a lot in most dishes and the amount of fat per serving is just about 4 grams, compared to around 30 grams in regular ground beef.

There are other alternatives. Many stores sell ultra-lean ground beef that has around 7 grams of fat per 4-ounce uncooked serving. There is also ground beef-style textured vegetable protein. This may not sound familiar to you, but anytime you eat imitation bacon bits, you are eating textured vegetable protein. It is a low-fat soy derivative that is indistinguishable from ground beef in sauces, soups and casseroles. Textured vegetable protein is sold in health food stores and mail order health related catalogs. It comes in other styles such as beef and chicken chunks, and the bacon bits we have all eaten. Unlike crunchy bacon bits, cooked textured vegetable protein develops the texture and taste of cooked meat, but with less fat and calories. You might want to give it a try.

You may notice that I don't include ground beef in many of my recipes that traditionally are made with it, for example, lasagna or tacos. I usually make these dishes without meat because we like them just as much without it. If you prefer it, by all means add some. Just be sure you use the ultra-lean kind and just a little of it.

SPICE IS THE VARIETY OF LIFE

The title may be a corny twist on the old saying, but it is the truth. Spices do add variety to life by enhancing the taste of food. Along with herbs and condiments, they are particularly important in adding flavor to low-fat dishes. They replace some of the sensory satisfaction usually provided by fat. My spice cabinet is overflowing with just about every spice and herb available. I like nothing more than adding a lot of them to my food. The amounts shown in my recipes are only guidelines. Keep adding a little at a time until the dish is as spicy as you like. I normally double or even triple the amount.

It is now possible to find almost any spice or herb in discount stores, where they often cost less than $1 per bottle. At that price, you may be able to afford to experiment. It's fun to make up some tasty spice and herb blends.

I also love to keep a lot of condiments on hand. Many of the sauces and other condiments in the grocery store are fat-free. If a dish seems bland, just add a dollop of catsup, a splash of hot sauce, or a spoonful of spicy relish. If you season your foods well with herbs, spices and condiments, you'll find that you don't miss the fat at all.

A Guide To Basic Spices

Allspice has a delicate, spicy flavor that resembles a blend of cloves, cinnamon and nutmeg. It is used in baked goods, preserves, relishes and puddings.

Anise has a sweet, licorice flavor. It is used in cakes, cookies, and sweet breads.

Basil has a mild taste. It is often used in tomato dishes, but is also good with peas, squash, green beans, salads and chicken.

Bay leaves have a rather sweet taste. They are often used in soups and stews.

Caraway seeds have a pronounced zesty taste with hints of dill. They are often used in sauerkraut, noodles and rye bread, but are also good with potatoes, green beans and carrots.

Chervil has flavor similar to parsley but milder. It is very popular in France. It is used in salads, sauces and soups.

Curry is a blend of many spices, among them ginger, turmeric, and fenugreek. It is commonly used in Indian dishes.

Dill has a clean, aromatic taste. It is widely used in pickling, but also adds flavor to sauerkraut, potatoes and macaroni dishes.

Fennel has a licorice flavor. It is used in many dishes, from salads and soups to cookies and cakes.

Ginger has a fresh, spicy flavor. It is used in meat, vegetable and dessert dishes.

Mace is very similar to nutmeg in flavor, which is understandable since it is the outer covering of the nutmeg seed. It is used in baked goods and pickling.

Marjoram has a sweet, minty flavor. It is used with lamb, and in soups and stews.

Mint has a mild flavor in spearmint and a stronger, peppery flavor in peppermint. Spearmint is used in sauces. Peppermint is most commonly used in candies and desserts. Mint also goes well with a few vegetables, such as potatoes and peas.

Mustard has a sharp, spicy flavor. Ground mustard is used to make one of our most popular condiments. Mustard seeds are used in sauerkraut and cabbage dishes.

Oregano is an aromatic, spicy herb often used in tomato dishes.

Parsley is very mild in flavor, with curly leaves that make it a popular garnish. Italian parsley has a flatter leaf and stronger flavor. It is often used in soups, casseroles, and vegetable dishes.

Paprika has a sweet, mild flavor. It is used to give color to pale foods, and as a seasoning in chicken dishes and salad dressing.

Poppy seeds are tiny, nutty tasting seeds that are found in baked goods and noodle dishes.

Rosemary has a sweet, fresh taste. It is popular in lamb dishes, and with potatoes, chicken and peas.

Sage has a rather minty flavor. It is used in stuffing, meat dishes and in sausage.

Tarragon has a licorice flavor. It is used in sauces, salads, vegetable dishes and chicken dishes.

Thyme has a strong flavor. It is used with poultry, fish and vegetable dishes.

Turmeric has a peppery flavor. It is used as a coloring and flavoring agent in pickles and mustard.

OIL SUBSTITUTES IN BAKED GOODS

People are amazed when they ask for my corn bread recipe and I list applesauce as one of the ingredients. They cannot believe that it doesn't make the finished product taste like a dessert. You actually can't taste it at all. It simply imparts a moistness that usually takes oil to achieve. Try using applesauce in any baked goods that you prepare, measure for measure.

In addition, there are other oil substitutes available that you might want to try. Fat-free sour cream and fat-free cottage cheese can also add moistness to baked goods, as can baby food prunes. You might like to experiment and find the one that works best for you.

Serving Suggestions For Fresh Fruit

I keep a variety of fresh fruits in case I want something sweet. It is very filling and much better for you than most desserts or snack foods. Most traditional desserts and commercially prepared snack foods just leave you hungry for more. That old advertising slogan for potato chips—"Bet you can't eat just one"—has a lot of truth in it. Eat one apple and you are full. Eat one piece of cake and you'll want another. If plain fresh fruit becomes boring, try some of my ideas for pepping it up.

1. Slice the fruit into thin wedges. Arrange attractively around a small mound of granulated sugar substitute mixed with a bit of cinnamon or nutmeg. Dip each bite of fruit into the mixture. You can also make a dip for the fruit by combining a little fat-free sour cream or yogurt with a dash of vanilla, some sugar substitute and cinnamon.

2. Prepare a small box of sugar-free vanilla pudding mix with skim milk, using a bit more than the package directions suggest. The pudding should be the consistency of a fairly thick sauce. Pour a small amount of the sauce over fruit.

3. Crumble a cinnamon-sugar graham cracker. Sprinkle over a bowl of cooked or uncooked fresh fruit. The effect is a little like fruit cobbler.

4. Make fat-free frozen yogurt a topping for fruit. Place a very small scoop of vanilla frozen yogurt atop a bowl of cooked or uncooked fruit. Allow it to soften slightly.

Low-fat Cooking Methods

How To Fry and Saute Foods the Low-fat Way

I always loved fried foods, but I hated to prepare them at home since cleaning an oil spattered stove top was not my idea of fun. Years ago, when I learned about oven frying, I was thrilled. I could enjoy fried foods without the mess or the constant attention that stove top frying requires.

Fortunately, oven frying adapts well to low-fat cooking techniques. I generally place a sheet of aluminum foil on a baking sheet with low sides. I then coat the foil with no-stick cooking spray. I also coat the food with the cooking spray after it has been placed on the baking sheet. This aids in browning. The cooking spray is primarily oil, so don't saturate the baking sheet or the food with it. The main benefit of using the spray instead of bottled oil is that a 1¼ second spritz, which is a sufficient amount to coat a 10" skillet, has less than 1 fat gram and only 7 calories, compared to 12-14 fat grams and 120 calories per tablespoon for bottled oil. If you prefer to use some of your fat grams to oven fry with bottled oil or even reduced-fat mayonnaise, see more of my tips for oven frying in the section entitled "Some Ideas For Oven Frying." One more thing I like about oven frying is that when you finish, the foil can be discarded. The baking sheet will seldom need washing.

You will also find no-stick cooking spray a great help in preparing sautéed foods. Just spray your skillet or sauté pan and add the vegetables or meat. I sometimes add a little bit of extra spray after the food has been placed in the pan. The spray comes in plain, butter and olive oil flavors, so you can impart the taste you prefer.

It is also possible to conventionally fry foods on the stove top using low-fat cooking techniques. You can quite successfully fry both breaded and unbreaded foods using either the cooking spray or by using just a tablespoon of oil.

One additional frying technique is the use of chicken broth! Place a tablespoon or so of defatted chicken broth in your skillet. Place the skillet over medium heat. When the broth begins to simmer, add your food. Because chicken broth evaporates, you may need to add an additional amount during the cooking process. Believe it or not, the foods, including fried chicken, will brown somewhat, although they will not be very crisp. The skillet needs to be well coated with no-stick cooking spray before the broth is added. Otherwise the breading may stick to the skillet. Chicken broth can also be used to sauté or to stir-fry.

Some Ideas For Oven Frying

I normally don't use any oil to oven fry, since I think that no-stick cooking spray does an acceptable job. However, you might prefer to use oil, tahini or reduced-fat mayonnaise. Remember that both vegetable oil and tahini have considerable fat grams. Most oils have 12-14 grams per tablespoon. Tahini, a delicious sesame seed paste found in health food stores and larger grocery stores, has about 8 fat grams per tablespoon. Reduced-fat mayonnaise has around 3-5 grams per tablespoon, depending upon the brand.

Sliced vegetables, chicken and fish are all candidates for oven frying. You might like to prepare them in the following quick and easy manner:

Place the vegetables or chicken in a zipper top plastic bag. Add 1 tablespoon oil, tahini or reduced-fat mayonnaise. Zip the bag and work the vegetables around so that each piece gets coated. Add ½ cup fine, dry breadcrumbs. Garlic powder, salt and pepper, or other spices may be added, according to preference. Bake the vegetables or chicken on a shallow baking sheet that has been sprayed with no-stick cooking spray at 425° until browned to your taste.

Outdoor Cooking

Who doesn't love the aroma and taste of foods cooked on an outdoor grill? Don't think that living a low-fat lifestyle will put a damper on your enjoyment of foods cooked outdoors. Chicken, beef top round, turkey, fish, lean pork tenderloin and even low-fat wieners are wonderful when grilled, barbecued or smoked. Even if fatty ribs have always been your meat of choice when cooking outdoors, you can make a reasonable facsimile by slicing pork tenderloins into thick strips that resemble the boneless country style ribs sold in the grocery store. Since the meats that you will be cooking are not fatty, you will need to be careful not to let them dry out. Reduced cooking temperature, carefully watched cooking time and use of marinades, or basting sauces can take care of that possibility. Here's another use for good old no-stick cooking spray: Coat the food to be cooked outdoors with no-stick spray. It will keep it from sticking to the grill, and will add a tiny bit of oil to the food, which will keep it more moist. Perfectly delicious grilled chicken can be prepared by simply coating boneless breasts with the spray, then sprinkling them with garlic powder and/or herbs to taste. If you also spray your grill rack, it will be easier to clean.

Vegetables are also terrific cooked outdoors, either combined with meat in a kabob or grilled whole or in slices along with the entrée. They may be wrapped in foil first, if desired. I personally like the vegetables cooked directly on the grill, so that they absorb more of the outdoor flavor. No-stick cooking spray, as well as garlic, herbs or basting sauces that enhance flavor, are terrific helps when cooking vegetables on the grill. So is the accessory grill rack made with smaller grids. It prevents small items like vegetable slices or shrimp from falling through.

Many traditional accompaniments to outdoor meals can be easily prepared in a low-fat manner. Baked beans, coleslaw and potato salad are delicious made the low-fat way. You may have other side dishes that you like to serve with your outdoor meals. With your imagination and the low-fat substitutes on the market, there is virtually no dish that you can't adapt to the low-fat lifestyle. That is part of the beauty of it!

BOUNTIFUL BEANS:
A GUIDE TO BEANS AND THEIR PREPARATION

I cannot say enough good things about beans. They have become just about my favorite food. They are a large part of my success on the low-fat lifestyle. They are easy to prepare, versatile, nutritious, and best of all, filling. When you make a bean dish a large part of your meal, you fill up quickly and stay full. While it is possible to find fresh beans at times, most of the time I depend on the dried version. In a pinch, canned beans will do. However, it is very inexpensive and easy to prepare dried beans yourself. I like to soak them overnight, then cook them all day in the slow cooker. When I come home from work, they are ready to eat. There are two basic ways to soak dried beans. Choose the one that best suits your schedule:

Overnight Method: Wash and pick over the beans. Cover one pound of beans with 6-8 cups of water. There are disagreements about cooking beans in the soaking water. Some nutritionists feel that they should be, so that nutrients removed in the soaking process will not be lost. Others feel that the nutrients lost are negligible, and that the soaking water should be replaced with fresh water. You can make your own choice. I prefer to discard the soaking liquid.

Quick soaking method: Place the beans, along with 6-8 cups of water per pound, in a kettle over medium heat. Bring to a rapid boil, remove from the heat, and let stand one hour. Then cook as usual. Beans may be cooked on the stovetop over medium heat, according to package directions, for 45 minutes to three hours, depending on the bean. They may also be cooked in a slow cooker for 8-12 hours on low. My favorite way to season dried beans is to add 1-2 chicken bouillon cubes for each two cups of water.

While most of us are familiar with common types of dried beans, here is a short guide in case you need it:

Black beans: A small, black, kidney shaped bean that is heavily used in Caribbean-style dishes, such as Cuban black beans. They are also called turtle beans.

Blackeyed peas are small and cream colored with a small, black mark at the sprouting point. They are also called cow peas. Because they are thin-skinned, they can be cooked without soaking.

Butter beans come in two varieties, the large butter bean and the smaller lima bean. Both are popular and delicious.

Chickpeas are also called garbanzo beans. They are probably most familiar as an ingredient at salad bars, but they are used in a large number of Mediterranean-style dishes. They are very nutritious, with high amounts of protein and B vitamins.

Northern and navy beans are very popular all over the world. In this country the navy bean is probably best known as the bean used in baked beans.

Kidney beans are large red beans that are probably best known for their role in Mexican-style dishes.

Lentils are thought to be the first beans to be eaten by man. There are several varieties. The most common variety is the brown lentil. They are very high in protein.

Peas are thought to go back to the days of ancient Rome. The most common variety is the English pea.

Pintos are among the most popular beans in this country. They are an important ingredient in many Mexican-style dishes.

Soy beans are eaten all over the world, but in this country are often used to create other products.

GLORIOUS GRAINS:
SOME OLD AND NEW GRAINS TO ENJOY

It is entirely appropriate that the bread, cereal, rice and pasta group makes up the broad, strong base of the food pyramid. All of these foods are grains in one form or another. Just as they are the foundation on which the pyramid rests, they are the foundation of my low-fat lifestyle. Grains are versatile, full of nutrients and fiber, and are wonderfully filling. Use them as a mainstay in your meals and you will not get hungry. While the old standbys, wheat, rice, oats and corn are most familiar and popular, more unusual grains, such as millet and bulgur, can add variety to your meals. For the adventurous, some ancient grains are becoming a modern day delicacy. Amaranth, quinoa and Job's Tears may delight you as much as they delighted people a thousand years ago. You may choose to enjoy your grains in their natural state or ground into flour and made into bread or pasta. However you eat them, they are sure to become a favorite part of your low-fat lifestyle.

While we may be unfamiliar with a number of the more obscure grains on the market, we often don't know much about the ones we've eaten all our lives. The following pages will give you a brief description of a number of grains, both common and uncommon. In addition, there is a chart which gives you the cooking instructions for many of them.

Before beginning a description of various grains and grain products, you should know what makes up a kernel of grain. It is actually a seed of the plant. The outer layer of the seed is called the husk, and it is removed from grains that are prepared for humans to eat. Inside the husk is the bran layer, which is high in fiber. The germ is also a nutritious part of the seed, full of protein, vitamins and minerals. The endosperm is the starchy center of the seed, and is the only part left in highly processed grain products. Since much of the nutrition of the grain is in the bran and germ, it is easy to see that the less the grain is processed, the better it is for us. Therefore, select as many whole-grain products as possible.

Amaranth is the ancient grain staple of the Aztecs. Amaranth is very different and may not be to everyone's taste. Amaranth and amaranth flour are available in health food stores.

Barley is mainly available in a form called pearl barley, which has had the hull and bran removed. It is often added to soups and stews, but is also excellent as a side dish with meals.

Buckwheat is mainly available ground into flour which is used in pancakes and bread, or as kasha, which is toasted buckwheat.

Bulgur is made from wheat berries that have been degermed, steamed and dried. It is often sold in medium and finely ground forms.

Cornmeal is basically ground, dried corn. It is commonly available in both white and yellow forms. Blue cornmeal is popular in some areas. Dried corn is also used to create other products. Hominy is dried corn that has been treated with lye or slaked lime, while grits are made from finely ground hominy. Masa harina is hominy that has been very finely ground. It is used to make corn tortillas.

Couscous is a grain product. Many people think of it as a grain, but it is made from durum wheat and is actually similar to pasta. It is very popular in Middle Eastern cooking.

Job's Tears is an interesting name for a unique grain that is popular in Asian countries. It resembles barley in many ways.

Millet, while not eaten much in this country, is a staple in many parts of the world. It consists of round, crunchy, yellow seeds and can be eaten cooked as a side dish or added to breads for textural interest.

Oats are a staple on many breakfast tables in the form of oatmeal, which is actually the steamed and rolled form of whole-grain oat groats. Most oatmeal is either whole rolled oat grains or rolled oats that have been cut up to make them cook more quickly. Unprocessed whole oat groats are also good when cooked and served as a side dish or included as an ingredient is breads.

Quinoa is the grain of the ancient Inca Indians. It is becoming quite popular in modern times, in part due to the very high nutritional value. It is available in health food stores.

White rice is rice that has been highly processed. Only the endosperm of the kernel is left. It is one of the most widely eaten grains.

Brown rice is not as popular as white rice. However it is somewhat more nutritious since the germ and bran have not been removed. Because of this, it has a chewier texture than white rice.

Rye is most widely available in this country in the form of flour, which is used as an ingredient in several breads, such as rye bread and pumpernickel.

Triticale is actually a hybrid grain made by crossing wheat with rye. It looks a little like rice. The nutritional value of triticale is very high.

Wheat is of course the queen of grains. The whole-wheat kernel is often sold as wheat berries which are eaten cooked as a cereal or side dish. They are also added to whole-wheat breads. Wheat berries are also often sprouted. Cracked wheat and bulgur are also forms of wheat which are quite popular. However, most wheat is ground into flour which is used to make breads, pastas and numerous other food products. Most are made with white flour, which is highly processed. It consists of the bleached, ground endosperm of the wheat kernel. Whole-wheat flour is less processed than white flour and therefore has more nutritional value. Products made with whole-wheat flour are also generally more filling and have more textural interest than those made with white flour.

Wild rice has always been viewed as a gourmet food, partly because it is very expensive. It is not a rice but the seed of a grass that grows in water. In recent years, it has become more widely available and is probably most popular with consumers when teamed with white or brown rice in packaged mixes.

A SHORT COURSE IN COOKING GRAINS

The following chart is for preparation of one cup of uncooked grain. The grain should be added when the water has come to a rolling boil. Allow the water to boil again, reduce the heat, cover tightly, and simmer for the number of minutes shown on the chart. It is usually best to allow the cooked grain to stand for a few minutes before serving. I generally do not add salt before cooking. After cooking, I use just a bit of light salt. The amount of salt shown on the chart is optional.

Grain	Water	Salt	Cooking Time	Yield
Barley	3 cups	1 teaspoon	40 min.	3 ½ cups
Buckwheat	2 cups	1 teaspoon	12 min.	3 ½ cups
Bulgur	2 cups	¼ teaspoon	20 min.	3 cups
Grits	4 cups	1 teaspoon	5 min.	4 cups
Millet	2 cups	½ teaspoon	30 min.	4 cups
Oat Groats	2 cups	½ teaspoon	60 min.	2 ½ cups
Oats Rolled	2 ¼ cups	½ teaspoon	7 min.	1 ½ cups
Oats, Quick	2 cups	¼ teaspoon	2 min.	1 ¼ cups
Rice, White	2 cups	1 teaspoon	20 min.	3 cups
Rice, Brown	2 ½ cups	1 teaspoon	45 min.	3 cups
Wheat Berries	2 ½ cups	½ teaspoon	2 hours	3 cups

HOW TO CAN HOMEMADE CONDIMENTS

Since I admittedly do not like to spend a lot of time in the kitchen, you may be surprised to see directions here for a time consuming task like home canning. Once in a blue moon I am overcome by a brief spell of domesticity. When this happens, I usually end up canning something, or making a loaf or two of homemade whole-grain bread. Condiments such as chow-chow, chutney and chili sauce can add a special zip to bean dishes, so I like to keep a variety on hand. While there are many good commercial brands on the market, it can be fun to create some gourmet chutneys, relishes or sauces at home. I had never canned a thing in my life until about a year ago. My husband and I were on vacation in a rustic mountain resort when we stumbled upon a gourmet food shop that specialized in unique homemade condiments. They averaged $5.00 per half pint. I decided that if they could do it, so could I. I purchased a few canning supplies and periodically, when I am in the mood, I put up a few jars of homemade chutney, relish or whatever else strikes my fancy, for us to enjoy with our meals. I usually can them rather than store them in the refrigerator or freezer. I do this because it keeps my freezer and refrigerator space free, and because I like to give a few jars to friends.

You may want to give home canning a try, too. It gives you a great feeling to look in the cupboard and see these lovely jars of gourmet treats that you have prepared yourself. You may enjoy making some of my favorite chutney and relish recipes. I have included them in the condiment section of this book. These recipes do call for quite a bit of sugar. However most people only eat a spoonful or two as an accompaniment, so the actual amount of sugar in a normal serving is quite small.

When home canning, it is very important to follow proper canning procedures. Otherwise, spoilage may occur. Never eat a canned food if the lid is bulging or if the food looks or smells like it may be spoiled. Do not use the following method to can meat or vegetables. They must be processed in a pressure canner. The boiling water bath method described here is used to process chutneys, relishes, pickles, fruits, tomatoes, jams and jellies.

You will need a kettle or pot deep enough to permit water to cover the tops of the canning jars by at least an inch. You will also need a rack, or insert that will hold the jars at least ½ inch above the bottom of the pot. It is essential to have a jar lifter to remove the hot jars from the water. You will also need pint or half pint canning jars, lids and bands that have been sterilized. This is done by pouring boiling water over them. Allow them to remain in the water so that they will still be hot when you are ready to use them. Use new canning jar lids and jars that have no cracks or chips.

Use only blemish-free, firm fruits and vegetables when preparing recipes for canning. While the chutney, relish or sauce is being cooked, bring sufficient water to a boil in your canning kettle to cover the tops of the filled jars by one inch. Allow room at the top so that the water will not boil over the sides of the kettle when the filled jars are placed in it. Pour the hot, cooked food into the hot, sterilized canning jars. Place the lids and seals on the jars. Place the filled jars in the boiling water. Allow enough room around each jar for free circulation of the water. If the water does not come at least one inch above the tops of the jars, add additional boiling water. Begin counting the processing time when the water returns to a full rolling boil. Keep the water boiling all during the processing period. Add additional boiling water if at any time the water boils down below the required height.

When the processing time ends, remove the jars from the kettle. Place the hot jars on a rack or on several thicknesses of cloth to cool. Do not put the jars on a cold surface or in a cold place or they may crack. After several hours test the seal by pressing down on the middle of the lid. If it will not move, the jar should be sealed. If it is not sealed, replace the lid with a new one and reprocess in the boiling water bath.

Don't be put off by the lengthy directions for processing canned condiments. It is really kind of fun and a few hours work will give you a lot of good things to eat, as well as save you money.

BASIC VEGETABLE COOKING

When we begin a low-fat lifestyle, we have to rethink our old cooking habits. I personally used to never prepare basic, cooked vegetables without several heaping tablespoons of butter. I just didn't think I could like them any other way. It is really all a matter of habit. When you get used to foods cooked without the butter or oil, you really begin to prefer them that way.

To prepare basic vegetables or legumes, add 1 chicken bouillon cube per 1-2 cups of cooking water. If you cannot do without a bit of butter or margarine, add 1 teaspoon to the recipe before serving. One way to get more bang for the buck, so to speak, if you must add butter, is to make browned butter. You simply melt real butter in a saucepan and cook over medium heat until the solids turn a rich brown. Watch carefully, since it can burn quickly. Remove the butter from the heat. As it cools, stir so that the solids are distributed throughout. Keep in the refrigerator and use a teaspoon or less only on those occasions when you feel that you must. The browned butter adds a delicious richness. A level teaspoon full has approximately 4 fat grams. I personally prefer to avoid any butter or margarine except for the ultra-light brands.

Remember, fat-free butter-flavored granules, sauces, spices or even plain catsup can give you much more taste than butter or margarine. If you want more seasoning in your basic vegetables, give them a try. Remember, butter, margarine and oil all have 12-14 fat grams per tablespoon. Butter should also be avoided if you have high cholesterol.

Oven roasting is a delicious way to prepare many vegetables. Simply cut them into chunks and place in a baking dish that has been sprayed with butter-flavored cooking spray. After the vegetables have been placed in the pan, spray them with the butter-flavored spray. Bake at 400° until the vegetables are tender and lightly browned.

Steaming is probably the most nutritious way to cook basic vegetables. See the steaming chart in this book for steaming methods and cooking times. Light soy sauce, liquefied butter-flavored granules, or even a light spray with butter-flavored cooking spray are quick and simple ways to season steamed vegetables.

Of course, another easy way to prepare many vegetables is to sauté or stir-fry them. Place them in a skillet or wok that has been sprayed with no-stick cooking spray and cook until done to your preference. A bit of chicken broth or water may also be added. Vegetables are often more tasty and retain more color and nutrients if they are served tender-crisp.

A SHORT GUIDE TO STEAMING

Steaming is a very nutritious way to prepare vegetables, chicken or seafood. It is also quick and easy. A simple, inexpensive insert that can turn any pot into a steamer can be purchased at almost any grocery or discount store for just a few dollars. For those who are willing to spend a little more for convenience, there are electric steamers which will steam a whole meal and then cut themselves off. Steaming allows the true taste of the food to shine, a fact that you will especially like as you decrease your dependence on fat and increase your appreciation of naturally good tasting food.

Basic steaming is simply a matter of suspending the food above boiling water so that the steam rising from the water cooks the food. As in other methods of cooking, timing is everything. A few extra minutes of steaming can change a tender-crisp stalk of asparagus into a sodden lump. Following is a general guide to the steaming times for some commonly steamed foods.

Artichokes: Choose blemish-free, compact artichokes. Trim off about an inch from the top, as well as the sharp tip from each leaf. Steaming time ranges from 30-45 minutes, depending on size.

Asparagus: Choose blemish-free, deep green, thin stalks. Break off the tough, woody end of each stalk. If the stalks are left whole, they will be tender-crisp in 8 minutes. If cut into pieces, it will take about 6 minutes.

Beans, Green: Choose blemish-free, crisp beans that snap easily. Remove the ends. Break into pieces or steam whole. Whole green beans will be tender-crisp in about 12 minutes. Beans that have been broken into pieces will take 10 minutes.

Beets: Choose deep red, firm beets with healthy green tops. Before steaming, cut off the tops, leaving about 2" of stem. Scrub the beets well. They will cook in 30-40 minutes.

Broccoli: Choose blemish-free, deep green stalks with no sign of yellow in the florets. Trim off the tough portion of the stalk. Cut into small pieces or steam whole. Broccoli will be tender-crisp in about 10-15 minutes.

Brussels Sprouts: Choose blemish-free, compact sprouts with no wilted leaves. Trim the ends and cut a small x in the base. They will steam in about 15 minutes.

Cabbage: Choose blemish-free, compact heads. Remove any wilted leaves and cut into wedges or shred. Shredded cabbage will steam in about 10 minutes, wedges will take about 15 minutes.

Carrots: Choose well-shaped, bright orange carrots. Peel them, using a vegetable peeler, and slice, or steam whole. Sliced carrots steam in about 10 minutes. Whole carrots take about 15-20 minutes.

Cauliflower: Choose compact, blemish-free heads. Trim away the outer leaves and cut into florets or steam whole. Florets will steam in 10-15 minutes. Whole heads will take about 15-20 minutes.

Chicken: Select boneless, skinless chicken breast halves. Trim away any remaining fat or skin. The steaming time will be 12-15 minutes.

Corn: Choose ears of corn with green, fresh looking husks. The kernels should be full and plump. Remove the husks and silk. An ear of corn steams in 8-10 minutes.

Eggplant: Choose blemish-free, deep purple eggplant. It can be steamed peeled or unpeeled, whole or in slices or cubes. Eggplant steams in 10-20 minutes, depending on whether it is cooked whole or cut into slices or cubes.

Fish fillets: Select fresh-smelling fillets of uniform thickness. Allow 10 minutes of steaming for each inch of thickness. If the fish is frozen, allow at least 20 minutes per inch.

Onions: Select blemish-free, firm onions. They may be peeled or steamed with the skin on. Steaming time will be about 15 minutes for sliced or chopped onions and 20 minutes for whole onions.

Peas, Green: Select peas with crisp, healthy pods. Sugar snap peas or snow peas should be steamed whole. Other green peas should be shelled shortly before steaming. Peas should steam for about 10 minutes.

Potatoes, Sweet: Choose plump potatoes with deep orange flesh. They may be steamed peeled or unpeeled, whole or in pieces. Whole sweet potatoes steam in about 25-40 minutes depending on size. Cut up sweet potatoes steam in 10-15 minutes.

Potatoes, White: Choose blemish-free, firm potatoes. They may be steamed peeled or unpeeled, whole or cut into pieces. Whole potatoes steam in 25-40 minutes. Potatoes cut up into slices or cubes should steam in about 20-30 minutes.

Rice, White or Brown: Add approximately 1½ cups water or chicken broth per cup of rice. Steam for about 40 minutes.

Shrimp: Choose fresh-looking peeled or unpeeled shrimp. Steam for about 11 minutes per pound. When they turn pink, they are done.

Spinach: Choose healthy, fresh-looking leaves. Remove any large or thick stems. Steam for 5-10 minutes.

Squash, Acorn: Choose heavy, dark green squash. Cut them in half and remove the strings and seeds. Place cut side down in the steaming basket. Steam for 25-30 minutes.

Squash, Summer: Choose blemish-free yellow squash or zucchini. Steam whole or cut into slices, for about 15 minutes.

Steamed vegetables, chicken and seafood are delicious alone or with very simple dressings, such as a squirt of lemon, a dash of soy sauce or a sprinkle of butter-flavored granules. A light sauce is also a good accompaniment.

Quick and Healthy Cooking the Microwave Way

Like steaming, microwaving is a particularly good way to prepare vegetables. Since little water is used, the vegetables retain their fresh, bright color and taste. They also lose fewer nutrients in the cooking process than vegetables boiled in water. As an added bonus, micro-waved foods can often be cooked and served in the same dish. In general, vegetables and other foods cooked in the microwave should be placed in covered, microwave-safe casserole dishes. Often the water that remains on them after washing is enough to cook them properly. Below is a short guide to microwaving vegetables and other common-ly microwaved foods. (The cooking times given are for 600-700 watt microwave ovens. Rotate the dish halfway through the cooking process.)

Artichokes: Wrap in waxed paper. Microwave on high 6-7 minutes per pound.

Asparagus: Arrange in a glass dish with 1 tablespoon water. Cover and microwave 6-7 minutes per pound on high.

Beans, Green: Place 3 cups green beans in a glass casserole. Add about ¼ cup water and microwave, covered, on high, for 8 minutes.

Corn: Remove the husks and silk and place the washed ears of corn in a covered dish or wrap in waxed paper with some of the water still clinging to them. Microwave on high 2-3 minutes for 1 ear, 6-7 min-utes for 4 ears or 10-12 minutes for 8 ears.

Eggplant: May be cooked peeled or unpeeled. Cut into cubes and microwave on high, covered, for 6-7 minutes per pound.

Fish: Place boneless fish fillets in a glass baking dish with the thick-er portions to the outside of the dish. Cover and microwave on medi-um power for 10 minutes per pound.

Greens: Place about 4 cups of washed greens in a casserole dish with the water still clinging to the leaves. Cover and microwave on high for 6-8 minutes.

Mushrooms: Clean the mushrooms and microwave whole or sliced in a covered glass dish on high for 6-7 minutes per pound.

Onions: May be left whole, sliced, or chopped. Microwave, covered, on high for 6-7 minutes per pound.

Peas, Green: Place 2 cups green peas in a casserole dish with 3 tablespoons water. Microwave, covered, on high for 5-6 minutes per pound. Stir halfway through the cooking time.

Beets: Place 2-4 beets in a glass casserole. Cover them with water and microwave on high, covered, for 15-18 minutes.

Broccoli: Arrange the stalks of broccoli with the stems pointing outward. Add 3-4 tablespoons water to the dish and cook, covered, on high for 8-10 minutes, depending on the size and number of stalks.

Cabbage: Shred, chop or slice into wedges. Place the cabbage in a glass cooking dish with 3 tablespoons water. Microwave on high, covered, for 7-8 minutes per pound.

Carrots: Slice carrots and place in a covered casserole with ¼ cup water. Microwave on high for 7-8 minutes per pound. Stir halfway through the cooking time.

Cauliflower: Leave whole or cut into florets. Add 3 tablespoons water to the cooking dish. Microwave, covered, on high for 6-7 minutes per pound. If the cauliflower has been cut into florets, stir halfway through the cooking time.

Chicken: Place boneless breast halves in a glass baking dish with the thicker parts to the outside of the dish. Cover and microwave on high for 4-5 minutes. Rearrange and turn the breasts and cook an additional 4-5 minutes.

Peppers: Place the washed, cored peppers in a glass baking dish. They may be sliced, chopped or left whole. Microwave, covered, on high for 6-7 minutes per pound.

Potatoes, Baked: Potatoes need to be similar in size and shape. Pierce skins. Arrange the potatoes in a circle in a baking dish, plate, or on the bottom of the oven. Microwave on high, 3-4 minutes for 1 potato, 6-7 minutes for two potatoes, 10-11 minutes for four potatoes.

Potatoes, Boiled: Peel and chop potatoes. Add about ½ cup water and microwave on high, covered, 18-20 minutes for four potatoes.

Potatoes, Sweet: Choose potatoes similar in size and shape. Arrange in a circle in a baking dish, on a plate, or on the bottom of the oven. Microwave on high 3-4 minutes for 1 potato, 5-6 minutes for two potatoes, 7-8 minutes for four potatoes, or 8-9 minutes for six potatoes.

Squash, Acorn: Pierce the whole squash in several places. Microwave 6-9 minutes on high. Let stand about 5 minutes, then cut in half and remove seeds.

Squash, Summer: Slice squash; place in a glass baking dish with 2 tablespoons water. Microwave, covered, on high for 6-7 minutes.

The Low-fat Kitchen

Kitchen Equipment For A Low-fat Lifestyle

Let's Go Grocery Shopping

KITCHEN EQUIPMENT FOR A LOW FAT LIFESTYLE

Good kitchen equipment can add enjoyment to the time you spend in the kitchen! Invest in the best you can afford.

Kitchen Basics:
Good quality nonstick cookware with tight fitting lids
Good quality nonstick bakeware
Good quality, sharp kitchen knives in assorted sizes
Mixing spoons, metal and wooden
Measuring spoons and cups
Metal and plastic colanders
A vegetable peeler
Strainers in several sizes
Wire whisks in several sizes
A spatula
A shredder/grater
A can opener
A kitchen scale
A cutting board

Helpful But not Essential Kitchen Equipment:
A blender
A food processor
An electric mixer
A garlic press
An instant reading thermometer
A slow cooker
A microwave oven
A steamer insert or bamboo steamer
A defatting cup
Kitchen shears
A pressure cooker
A wok
A waffle iron
A crepe skillet
A mini chopper
Microwaveable dishes

Kitchen Luxuries:
A Belgian waffle maker
An electric tortilla maker
An electric crepe maker
A pizza stone
An electric pasta maker
An electric bread maker
A grain mill
A wide slot toaster
An indoor electric grill
A convection oven
An air popcorn popper
An electric juicer
An ice cream maker
A pepper mill
A milkshake maker

LET'S GO GROCERY SHOPPING

Grocery shopping can be a lot of fun when you see all of the new low-fat products that come out weekly! The following is a general guideline to low-fat grocery shopping. Don't faint! You don't have to buy all of it! My best shopping tip: READ ALL NUTRITION LABELS! Make sure the goods you are buying are low-fat.

The Canned Goods section:
Any canned vegetable
Any canned water or juice-packed fruit
Fat-free spaghetti sauce
Canned Chinese vegetables, including water chestnuts
Canned dried beans
Canned tomatoes, tomato sauce and tomato paste (low sodium)
Canned fish, such as tuna, packed in water
Canned white chicken chunks, packed in water
Canned vegetable and fruit juices
Canned Mexican foods, such as chilies and fat-free refried beans
Canned evaporated skim milk
Canned baked beans
Canned 99% fat-free soups

Pasta, Grains, Beans, and Related:
White and brown rice
Noodles in various sizes, egg-free if possible
Gourmet rice, such as basmati and arborio
Instant rice
Packaged rice mixes and sauce mixes, low-fat
Packaged noodle and sauce mixes, low-fat
Dried beans of all kinds
Dried bean soup mixes
Barley
Assorted grains, such as oat groats, millet and bulgur
Instant mashed potatoes
Packaged potato and sauce mixes, low-fat
Packaged stuffing mix, low-fat

Breads, Crackers and Cookies:
Fat-free crackers
Fat-free rice cakes
Whole-grain crisp breads
Whole-grain reduced-calorie breads, rolls and buns
English muffins, assorted flavors
Bagels, assorted flavors
Pita bread
Melba toast
Fat-free and low-fat cookies
Fat-free croutons

Beverages:
Coffee, regular and assorted gourmet flavors
Tea, regular, and assorted flavored tea, regular and herbal
Diet hot cocoa mix (25 calories per cup)
Diet hot cider mix
Sugar-free powdered drink mixes
Diet soda

Baking Supplies:
White and whole-wheat flour (plain and self-rising)
Cornmeal
Buttermilk cornmeal mix
Fat-free baking mix
Yeast (rapid rise and regular)
Cocoa
Baking powder and baking soda
Dried skim milk powder

Cereals:
Rolled oats
Quick cooking oatmeal
Bran cereal
Fat-free or low-fat, low-sugar breakfast cereals
Grits

Cooking oils:
No-stick butter-flavored spray
No-stick olive oil-flavored spray
No-stick spray, unflavored
Small bottle olive oil
Small bottle canola oil

Packaged Dessert Mixes:
Sugar-free gelatin
Sugar-free pudding mix
Light cake mixes
Light frosting

Spices, Condiments and Related:
Louisiana hot sauce
Assorted mustards
Catsup (low sodium if possible)
Fat-free barbecue sauce
Worcestershire sauce
Liquid smoke

Fat-free and reduced-fat mayonnaise
Fat- free mayonnaise-type salad dressing
Fat-free salad dressing, assorted flavors
Pickles and pickle relish
Assorted vinegars
Imitation bacon bits
Light soy sauce
Light teriyaki sauce
Light salt
Coarse ground black pepper and whole peppercorns
Assorted spices and herbs
Salt-free spice blends
Salt substitute
Fat-free butter-flavor granules, in both package and shaker

The Meat Department:
Chicken pieces or boneless breasts (remove all skin and fat)
Whole turkey breast (remove skin)
Ultra-lean ground beef or butcher ground top round
97% fat-free wieners
Eye of round beef roast (all fat removed)
Pork tenderloin (all fat removed)
99% fat-free precooked turkey
98% fat-free precooked ham
Deli sliced 99% fat-free turkey
Deli sliced 98% fat-free ham
Fresh shrimp and other shellfish
Fresh fish fillets

Soups:
99% fat-free canned soups
Dehydrated soup mixes, including onion and vegetable
Bouillon cubes, chicken, vegetable, and beef (low sodium)
Instant bouillon granules, chicken and beef (low sodium)

The Dairy Case:
Fat-free egg substitute
Ultra-low-fat or fat-free margarine
Fat-free cream cheese
Fat-free hard cheeses, such as Cheddar and mozzarella
Fat-free sour cream
Fat-free yogurt
Skim milk
Fresh pasta
Fresh pasta sauces (fat-free)
Low-fat canned biscuits
Fresh refrigerated corn and flour tortillas

Frozen Foods:
Plain frozen vegetables
Frozen fat-free and low-fat dinners and entrées
Frozen pancakes
Frozen waffles (regular and Belgian)
Frozen sugar-free fruits
Frozen bread and roll dough
Frozen yogurt
Ice milk
Sherbet
Frozen juice bars

Produce:
Any fresh fruit, except avocado
Any fresh vegetable

Snack Foods:
Fat-free potato chips and corn chips
Popcorn (regular and low-fat microwave)
Fat-free dips
Pretzels

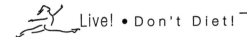

Miscellaneous:
Jelly, jams, and preserves-low or no-sugar brands preferred
Light pancake syrup, maple flavor
Light pancake syrup, blueberry flavor
Light chocolate sauce

The Low-fat Recipes That Helped Me Lose

Breakfast Foods

Appetizers and Snacks

Breads

Soups and Stews

Salads

Main Dishes

Vegetables

Grains and Pasta

The Fast Food Lover's Low-fat Path To Happiness

Desserts

Sauces and Condiments

Miscellaneous

Just A Few More Words About low-fat Recipes

On the following pages are the recipes that are a part of my low-fat lifestyle. Many are adaptations of recipes I used before I began counting fat grams. It is so simple to adapt recipes. Just replace the high-fat ingredients with low-fat alternatives. I have no trouble sticking with a low-fat lifestyle because I can enjoy most of my old favorites, with just a few modifications.

I am not a person who likes to spend a lot of time in the kitchen. As a matter of fact, the less time, the better. My recipes reflect that. They are short and uncomplicated. You may want to prepare more challenging recipes than I present here. If so, visit your local bookstore. There are a lot of cookbooks devoted to more sophisticated low-fat recipes. That is one thing I love about the low-fat lifestyle. Many conventional diets assume that people with weight problems love to cook and think about food all of the time. They believe that they must keep you busy cooking, weighing and measuring so that you won't notice that you are hungry. On a low-fat lifestyle you can have it either way. If you hate to cook, you fix it quick and get out of the kitchen. If you love to cook, you can find low-fat recipes that will make the most demanding gourmet happy.

Whether you love to cook or hate it, I imagine that you despise cleaning up afterwards. Everyone does. One great bonus of a low-fat lifestyle is that none of your dirty dishes will have the horrible greasy residue that is so hard to scrub off dishes in which fatty foods have been cooked or eaten. Is this a terrific lifestyle or what? Lots of great food to eat and dishes that are easier to clean, too!

You may notice that I list the number of fat grams, but not the calorie count per serving for each of my recipes. I do this because of my own experience. It is hard to forget about counting calories when you see them attached to every recipe.

When you prepare any of the recipes in this book, do not hesitate to modify them to your own taste. You may find that you prefer more or less herbs or spices. You might want to throw in a few extra low-fat ingredients. You may want to use some of your daily fat gram allowance to sauté or oven fry in a tablespoon of oil instead of using only the no-stick cooking spray that is suggested in a recipe. Please do not just take one taste of any low-fat dish or product and dismiss it just because it doesn't taste just like you think it should. Tinker with it if you must, but, above all, do not forget our words to live by: I WILL NOT LET MYSELF COMPARE THE TASTE OF MY LOW-FAT FOODS TO THEIR HIGH-FAT COUNTERPARTS. I WILL SIMPLY ENJOY THEM, WITHOUT MAKING ANY COMPARISON. You will come to love the taste of your low-fat dishes. After all, they can help you lose weight without dieting or deprivation.

BREAKFAST FOODS

I never skip breakfast! It gets my body cranked up in the morning! My personal favorites are oatmeal with sugar substitute, spices and/or fruit, pancakes with reduced-calorie syrup, or whole-grain toast with jam. I sometimes also throw in a bowl of cereal, an English muffin or a bagel if I am really hungry. If you are a bacon and eggs type person, you may decide to enjoy biscuits, several slices of low-fat precooked ham and scrambled eggs made with fat-free egg substitute or egg whites.

French Toast

½ cup fat-free egg substitute
½ cup skim milk
⅛ teaspoon nutmeg
1 teaspoon sugar or granular sugar substitute
fat-free, reduced-calorie bread slices
butter-flavored no-stick cooking spray

Combine the egg substitute, milk, nutmeg and sugar or sugar substitute. Cut the bread slices in half. Dip the bread into the egg mixture and sauté until golden on a griddle that has been sprayed with butter-flavor no-stick cooking spray. Good with light syrup, preserves or fruit sauce.

4 servings
0 fat grams per serving

Homemade Pancakes

I usually make pancakes with fat-free baking mix, or I buy the frozen ones at the grocery that are quite low in fat. However, when I have the time and inclination, I make them from scratch.

2 cups all-purpose flour
4 teaspoons baking powder
1 teaspoon light salt
1½ cups skim milk
¼ cup fat-free egg substitute
4 tablespoons fat-free cottage cheese
butter-flavored no-stick cooking spray

Combine the dry ingredients. In another bowl, combine the milk, egg substitute and the cottage cheese. Combine with the flour mixture. Cook the pancakes on a griddle that has been coated with butter-flavor no-stick cooking spray.

Variation: Add blueberries or sliced bananas to the batter.

4 servings
Less than 1 fat gram per serving

TERRIFIC OATMEAL

Frankly, oatmeal has probably done more to help me lose weight than anything else. Before I started following a low-fat lifestyle, I didn't eat oatmeal once a year. I didn't even particularly like it. Now I love it. I eat it often for breakfast. It also makes a great snack. It is healthy, wonderfully filling, and very versatile. Some people like it plain or with milk. I personally like to doctor it with lots or fruit, sugar substitute, and butter-flavored granules. Prepared this way, it becomes almost a dessert. With raisins and nutmeg, it is a little like rice pudding. With chopped peaches or apple it is tastes rather like fruit cobbler. I have even added a bit of cocoa powder! The results were not unlike a rich, fudgy dessert. Oatmeal has become one of my favorite comfort foods.

My Favorite Breakfast and Snack Oatmeal

Prepare as much quick cooking plain oatmeal as desired, according to the directions on the package. Add sugar substitute or sugar to taste. Blend in a sprinkle of nutmeg or cinnamon. Top with a sprinkling of butter-flavored granules and granular sugar substitute or sugar. Add raisins, cooked apple, or other fruit, if desired. A dash of vanilla, maple, or coconut flavoring instead of the spices is also terrific.

Approximately 2 fat grams
per cup of prepared oatmeal

APPETIZERS AND SNACKS

Appetizers and snacks can take the edge off hunger. However, they can also slow down your weight loss efforts if you overindulge. I could eat an entire family-size bag of fat-free tortilla chips and a whole recipe of dip by myself, so I try to save most traditional snack foods for an occasional treat. If I get hungry between meals, I most often have a piece of fruit, a bowl of oatmeal, or a cup of diet hot cocoa. Whole-grain reduced-calorie toast with jam also makes a filling snack.

Buffalo Chicken Breasts

This is a less fatty version of popular Buffalo Chicken Wings. For an authentic Buffalo Wings experience, serve with celery sticks and a small container of fat-free blue cheese dressing.

4 4-ounce chicken breast halves, boned and skinned
no-stick cooking spray
1 tablespoon melted margarine
1 tablespoon water
Louisiana hot sauce to taste

Cut the chicken breasts into strips, if serving as an appetizer, or leave whole to serve as an entrée. Sauté the chicken until brown in a skillet that has been coated with no-stick cooking spray. Combine the margarine, water and hot sauce. Add to the chicken in the skillet and simmer briefly.

4 servings
7 fat grams per serving

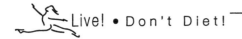

"Beanuts"

One day I happened to taste some raw chickpeas that had been soaked overnight in preparation for cooking. The flavor was very similar to that old southern favorite—boiled peanuts. I decided that the chickpeas might also taste good roasted. Since roasted peanuts are high in fat, these make a great substitute. Other dry beans may be substituted for the chickpeas.

2 cups dried chickpeas, soaked overnight/drained well

Arrange the chickpeas in a single layer on a baking sheet with low sides. Bake for about 40 minutes at 350°, stirring occasionally.

4 servings
2 fat grams per serving

Hummus

This is a popular dip that is delicious with toasted pita chips. Tahini (sesame seed paste), is quite high in fat, but the amount used in this recipe is not enough to blow your fat gram allowance.

1 16-ounce can chickpeas
1 tablespoon tahini (sesame seed paste)
2 tablespoons fresh lemon juice
2 cloves garlic, minced, or ¼ teaspoons garlic powder

Combine all of the ingredients in a food processor and puree.

8 servings
Less than 2 fat grams per serving

Lasagna Chips
1 8-ounce package lasagna noodles, cooked as directed
    on package
butter-flavored no-stick cooking spray
light salt
1 tablespoon grated Parmesan cheese

Cut the cooked noodles into 1" lengths. Place on a baking sheet that has been coated with butter-flavored no-stick cooking spray. Lightly coat the noodles with cooking spray. Sprinkle the noodles with salt and Parmesan cheese. Bake at 400° for about 15 minutes, or until brown. Heated spaghetti sauce makes a good dip with the chips.

6 fat grams in recipe

Lively Horseradish Dip
1 1-ounce envelope dehydrated onion soup mix
1 tablespoon imitation bacon bits
1 cup fat-free sour cream
horseradish to taste

Combine onion soup mix, imitation bacon bits, sour cream, and horseradish. Serve with fat-free chips, crackers, or crudities.

1 fat gram per serving

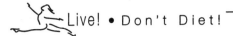

Mexican Bean Dip

2 cups cooked pinto beans or black beans, mashed
½ teaspoon garlic powder
1 can chopped chili peppers, drained
½ green pepper, chopped
½ medium onion, chopped
½ teaspoon cumin
hot sauce to taste

Combine the beans, garlic powder, chili peppers, green peppers, onion, cumin and hot sauce. Serve with baked tortilla chips

6 servings
0 fat grams per serving

Middle Eastern Eggplant Dip

1 medium eggplant
1 tablespoon tahini
2 cloves garlic, minced, or ¼ teaspoon garlic powder

Place the eggplant in a 375° oven and roast until the skin is charred. Let cool, cut in half, and remove the pulp. Mash the pulp and combine with the remaining ingredients. Serve with pita bread or toasted pita chips.

8 servings
1 fat gram per serving

Pineapple Cheese Spread
This recipe sounds just awful, but it is really good.

1 8-ounce container fat-free cream cheese, softened
1 8-ounce can crushed pineapple in its own juice,
    drained
2 tablespoons finely minced onion
2 tablespoons finely minced green pepper

Combine the softened cream cheese and the drained pineapple. Stir in the onion and the green pepper. Place the mixture in a small serving dish. Serve with fat-free snack crackers.

0 fat grams in the recipe

Sort of Guacamole
Since avocado is relatively high in fat, this recipe lets us have a guacamole-style dip without the avocado found in the traditional recipe. Serve with baked tortilla chips.

2 10-ounce packages frozen English peas, thawed
½ cup fat-free sour cream
1 small onion, finely minced
½ teaspoon dried cilantro
1 chopped tomato
½ teaspoon cumin

Puree the peas in a blender or food processor until smooth. Add the remaining ingredients. Serve chilled or at room temperature.

8 servings
0 fat grams per serving

BREADS

Breads are among the "Big Five" foods in my low-fat lifestyle. Along with beans, grains, fruits and vegetables, breads will fill you up and keep you satisfied. Whole-grain breads are the most nutritious and most filling, so choose them often.

Baked Hushpuppies

½ cup cornmeal
½ cup all-purpose flour
½ teaspoon sugar or granulated sugar substitute
½ teaspoon light salt
dash of ground red pepper
⅓ cup skim milk
¼ cup fat-free egg substitute
2 tablespoons fat-free sour cream
1 medium onion, finely minced

Combine the dry ingredients. Add the milk, egg substitute and sour cream. Mix in the onion. Bake in regular muffin tins, or mini tins, if you want them to be more like a traditional hushpuppy. Bake at 400° for 15-25 minutes, depending on the size of the muffin tins.

Less than 1 fat gram per muffin

Broccoli Cornbread

1 cup self-rising cornmeal mix
¼ cup fat-free egg substitute
½ cup water, or more if needed
½ cup fat-free cottage cheese
1 onion, chopped
1 10-ounce package frozen chopped broccoli,
    cooked and drained

Combine all of the ingredients. Pour into and 8" x 11.5" baking pan. Bake at 375° for 30-40 minutes.

8 servings
Less than 1 fat gram per serving

Cheese, Onion and Poppy Seed Dinner Bread

2 cups fat-free baking mix
1 medium onion, finely minced
¼ cup fat-free egg substitute
¾ cup water
4 ounces fat-free Cheddar cheese
1 tablespoon poppy seeds
1 tablespoon fat-free cottage cheese

Combine all of the ingredients. Pour into an 8" square baking pan. Top with a sprinkle of extra poppy seeds if desired. Bake at 400° for 20 minutes.

6 servings
Less than 1 fat gram per serving

Cinnamon Rolls

Since these contain sugar, they should be eaten only as a special treat. Too much sugar can hurt weight loss.

3 cups fat-free baking mix
¾ cup skim milk
¼ cup sugar
2 teaspoons cinnamon
butter-flavored no-stick cooking spray
¼ cup raisins
¼ cup powdered sugar mixed with 2 teaspoons skim milk

Combine the baking mix and the skim milk. Turn the dough out onto a flat surface that has been sprinkled with flour or baking mix. Roll the dough out into a 12" x 14" rectangle. Combine the sugar and cinnamon. Spray the dough with the cooking spray. Sprinkle the sugar-cinnamon mixture, then the raisins over the dough. Roll the dough up, beginning with the 14" side. Press the seam to help seal. Cut the roll into 12 1" pieces. Place in a 9" x 13" baking dish that has been sprayed with butter-flavored no-stick cooking spray. Bake for 25 minutes at 350°. Drizzle the powdered sugar mixture over the cinnamon rolls.

12 servings
0 fat grams per serving

Country Biscuits

A friend gave me this recipe long before I started watching fat grams. Luckily, they are low in fat so I didn't have to give them up. They are great served with fat-free margarine and reduced-sugar jam. You can even make a reasonable facsimile of the fast food chain favorite, breakfast in a biscuit, by adding a slice of 98% fat-free cooked ham and a scrambled egg made with fat-free egg substitute.

1 cup self-rising flour
1 tablespoon solid vegetable shortening
½ cup buttermilk
butter-flavored no-stick cooking spray

Cut the shortening into the flour, using a pastry blender or two knives. When completely blended, add the buttermilk. Roll out and use a biscuit cutter to cut into 8-10 biscuits. Place on a baking sheet that has been coated with butter-flavored no-stick cooking spray. After the biscuits have all been placed in the pan, spray the tops lightly with the butter-flavor spray. Bake at 425 for 10 minutes or until lightly browned.

8-10 servings
Less than 2 fat grams per serving

Our Daily Corn Bread

Okay, so it's not our daily corn bread, but I couldn't resist the pun. However, we do have it at least 3-4 times a week. My husband and I usually eat half the recipe each! I bake it in an 8" iron skillet that has been coated with no-stick cooking spray. We like it left in the oven for a long time, so that the outside becomes very crusty. This is especially good with dry beans. The onions and peppers are entirely optional. The corn bread is just as good without them. However, I like to add them because it doubles the size of the corn bread, while adding a lot of taste and no additional fat grams.

1 cup self-rising cornmeal mix
¼ cup fat-free egg substitute
½ cup water, or more for a thinner batter
¼ cup unsweetened applesauce
1 onion, chopped
1 green pepper chopped
no-stick cooking spray

Preheat the oven to 450°. Combine the cornmeal mix, egg substitute, water and applesauce. Add the onion and green pepper. Pour into an 8" skillet that has been coated with no-stick cooking spray. Bake for 30-45 minutes, depending upon how crisp you like the crust.

4 servings
1 fat gram per serving

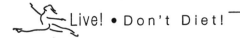

Stuffed Bread

I do not make a habit of keeping this around the house because it is entirely too tempting to me. It is nice for a special treat, however.

butter-flavored no-stick spray
1 pound loaf frozen bread dough, thawed

Roll dough into a 9"x 12" rectangle, spray with butter-flavored no-stick cooking spray, and sprinkle with one of the following fillings. Then roll up and place in a loaf pan. Let rise and bake according to the directions on the bread dough label.

Double onion filling:
1 1-ounce package dehydrated onion soup mix,
½ medium onion, finely chopped, ⅛ teaspoon poppy
seeds

Apple-cinnamon filling:
¼ cup brown sugar substitute, 2 apples, peeled and grated, 1 teaspoon cinnamon

16 servings
1 fat gram per slice

Tasty Dinner Bread

Sometimes a meal just cries out for some special, delicious bread as an accompaniment. Who can eat pasta without a few slices of warm garlic bread? If you think you can't prepare it without lots of butter, think again. I personally like to reserve my daily fat gram allowance for things other than 12 grams per tablespoon butter or margarine, so I prefer one of the following methods of making the bread without the fat:

Method 1: Use fat-free, reduced-calorie Italian or sourdough bread. Spray each slice lightly with butter-flavored no-stick cooking spray. Sprinkle with garlic powder and dried oregano. Bake at 350° until just warm, or until brown and crisp, depending on your personal preference.

Method 2: Use fat-free, reduced-calorie Italian or sourdough bread. Spread with a teaspoon of ultra-low-fat (2 grams per tablespoon or less) margarine. Sprinkle with garlic powder and dried oregano. Bake at 350° until warm or crisp depending on your preference.

Variation: Poppy seeds and dehydrated onion are also tasty additions.

Less than 1 fat gram per slice

SOUPS AND STEWS

Make a lot of these for a warm, satisfied feeling. I make several pots of Twelve Bean or Northern Bean soup every week, often in the slow cooker. A hearty soup or stew, served with corn bread or whole-grain bread and a salad, makes a wonderful meal. I often eat three large bowls of soup at a time.

Baked Bean Soup

3 16-ounce cans fat-free vegetarian baked beans,
    undrained
1 16-ounce can chopped tomatoes, undrained
3 97% fat-free wieners, sliced
1 medium onion, finely chopped
1 green pepper, finely chopped
1 tablespoon granulated brown sugar substitute
1 teaspoon prepared mustard

Combine all ingredients. Simmer until the onion and green pepper are tender.

6 servings
Less than 1 fat gram per serving

Chili

You may think if it doesn't have meat, then it's not chili, but it's still really good. You don't really miss the meat.

1 pound dry kidney beans
8 cups water
2 large onions, chopped
2 green peppers, chopped
2 15-ounce cans chunky Mexican-style tomato sauce
1 tablespoon chili powder
1 tablespoon cumin

Soak the beans overnight. Pour off the soaking water and replace with 8 cups fresh water. Cook the beans, onion and peppers for 1½ hours, or until tender. Add the tomato sauce, chili powder and cumin.

Variation: Add 6 ounces cooked ultra-lean ground beef or ½ cup dehydrated ground beef-style textured vegetable protein.

We like this chili with chopped onion and fat-free shredded Cheddar cheese on top.

6 servings
Less than 1 fat gram without meat

Cozy Corn Chowder

While a big steaming bowl of this tasty and filling chowder would be good any time of year, somehow it evokes thoughts of crisp fall days, red and gold leaves and football games. It would be just the thing to warm you up after a brisk day outdoors.

1 medium onion, minced
½ cup celery, minced
no-stick cooking spray
1 tablespoon all-purpose flour
2½ cups skim milk
1 ½-ounce package butter-flavored granules
1 17-ounce can creamed corn
2 medium potatoes, peeled and diced
8 ounces cooked 98% fat-free ham
light salt and pepper to taste

Sauté the onion and celery in a saucepan that has been coated with no-stick cooking spray. When they are wilted, add the flour and cook 1 minute. Gradually add the milk and stir until thickened. Add the butter-flavored granules, corn, potatoes, ham, salt and pepper. Simmer 20 minutes.

4 servings
2 fat grams per serving

Cream of Broccoli Soup

Since broccoli is supposed to be so good for us, we are supposed to eat lots of it, as often as possible. This is a good way to serve it.

2 cups water
1½ pounds fresh broccoli, chopped
½ cup onion
½ cup celery
2 tablespoons all-purpose flour blended with 2 tablespoons water
2½ cups water
½ cup evaporated skim milk
1 tablespoon chicken-flavor instant bouillon granules
salt and pepper to taste

Heat 2 cups of water until boiling. Add the vegetables and cook until tender. Purée half of the vegetables in the blender, along with the cooking liquid. Return the puréed vegetables to the cooking pot. Add the flour mixed with 2 tablespoons water. Stir until blended. Add the remaining 2½ cups of water, the evaporated skim milk and the bouillon granules. Bring to a boil and then simmer until slightly thickened. Add the remaining vegetables and continue cooking for 10 minutes.

9 cups
0 fat grams per serving

Northern Bean Soup

This is another regular on our menu. I love it because it, like most dishes made with dry beans, can cook all day in the slow cooker and be ready to serve when you get home from work.

1 pound dried northern beans, soaked overnight
8 cups water
3 medium potatoes, peeled and diced
2 carrots, peeled and sliced
1 cup celery, diced
8 ounces 98% fat-free precooked ham, cut into cubes
3 chicken bouillon cubes

After soaking the beans overnight, discard the soaking liquid. Add 8 cups fresh water and the rest of the ingredients. Cook up to 12 hours on low in a slow cooker or cook on medium heat for about 2 hours or until the vegetables are tender.

6 servings
2 fat grams per serving

Quick and Hearty Potato Soup

½ cup chopped onion
½ cup chopped celery
½ cup chopped carrots
no-stick cooking spray
6 cups skim milk
4 teaspoons chicken-flavor instant bouillon granules
2 medium potatoes, diced
1¾ cup instant mashed potato flakes

Sauté the onion, celery and carrots in a large saucepan that has been coated with no-stick cooking spray. When they are wilted, stir in the milk and the bouillon granules. Add the potatoes. Cook 8 minutes, stirring frequently. Add the potato flakes and cook 6 more minutes.

6 servings
Less than 1 fat gram per serving

Twelve Bean Soup Mix

Mix equal amounts of the following dry beans:

black beans	large lima beans	northern beans
pinto beans	split peas	field peas
kidney beans	baby limas	black-eyed peas
chickpeas	lentils	navy beans

It is a good idea to buy a pound of each of the beans and after mixing, store in a large container and remove as needed. It's much cheaper than buying the commercial multi-bean soup mixes.

To make 4-6 servings, soak 1½ cups of the mixed beans overnight. Discard the soaking water and replace with 8 cups of fresh water. Add 3 chicken bouillon cubes. Cook up to 12 hours on low in a slow cooker or simmer for 2½ hours on the stovetop. When the beans are done, mix them with the following:

1 15-ounce can mixed tomatoes and chilies
1 chopped onion
1 clove garlic, minced
salt and pepper to taste

Continue cooking for 30-40 additional minutes.

Less than 1 fat gram per serving

SALADS

A tasty salad can add interest to a meal and take the edge off your appetite! I keep a lot of assorted salad ingredients. They make great in-between-meal snacks, in addition to their usual role as a mealtime accompaniment or main dish. While I have prepared my own dressings on occasion, I usually buy a variety of the excellent fat-free dressings available at the market. Thousand Island, Ranch, Italian, French and Honey Mustard fat-free dressings can not only perk up a salad, or plain sliced fresh vegetables, they can also double as marinades and sandwich spreads. Fat-free mayonnaise can also benefit from the addition of a little fat-free salad dressing for a special taste.

Blueberry Salad

This could also double as a dessert.

1 6-ounce package sugar-free black cherry gelatin
2 cups hot water
1 15-ounce can crushed pineapple, juice-pack, drained
1 15-ounce can blueberries, drained

Dissolve the gelatin in hot water. Add pineapple and blueberries. Place in the refrigerator until jelled. Spread with the topping.

Topping:
4 ounces fat-free sour cream
4 ounces fat-free cream cheese
1 teaspoon vanilla
3 tablespoons sugar or granulated sugar substitute

Combine the topping ingredients. Spread on the gelatin layer.

8 servings
0 fat grams per serving

Carrot and Raisin Salad

5 cups shredded carrots

1 8-ounce can crushed pineapple (in its own juice),
    drained

¼ cup raisins

4 tablespoons reduced-fat mayonnaise (3 grams per
    tablespoon brand)

Combine all of the ingredients. Chill before serving.

5 servings
Less than 2 fat grams per serving

Chef's Salad

1 head iceberg lettuce, shredded

1 onion, thinly sliced

1 tomato, chopped

8 radishes, thinly sliced

1 cucumber, thinly sliced

8 ounces 98% fat-free precooked ham, cut into match-
    stick size pieces

4 hard boiled eggs, whites only, chopped

4 ounces fat-free Cheddar cheese, shredded

fat-free salad dressing

Place a layer of the shredded lettuce on a dinner plate, followed by layers of each of the other vegetables. Top with a portion of the ham, egg whites and the cheese. Add your favorite
fat-free dressing. Serve with fat-free crackers.

4 servings
2 fat grams per serving

"Couldn't Be Better For You" Salad

1 small cauliflower, chopped
1 bunch broccoli, chopped
1 bunch green onions, chopped
4 ounces fat-free Cheddar cheese, shredded
1 bottle fat-free Ranch salad dressing

Combine all ingredients and chill.

8 servings
0 fat grams per serving

Crisp Corn Salad

3 cans whole kernel corn, drained
1 cucumber, chopped
1 green pepper, chopped
1 small onion, chopped
3 fresh tomatoes, chopped
1 cup fat-free Italian salad dressing

Combine all ingredients. Serve cold.

6 servings
0 fat grams

Crispy Slaw
Slaw:
1 head cabbage, shredded
1 carrot, shredded
1 onion, finely chopped
1 green pepper, finely chopped

Dressing:
2 packets sugar substitute
4 tablespoons vinegar
4 tablespoons evaporated skim milk
½ teaspoon dry mustard
3 tablespoons fat-free mayonnaise
light salt and pepper to taste

Combine the slaw ingredients. In a separate container, mix the dressing ingredients. Combine the slaw and dressing.

8 servings
0 fat grams per serving

Deluxe Fruit Salad Bowl
4 navel oranges, peeled and sectioned
1 cup strawberries, halved
2 bananas, sliced
1 cup seedless grapes
½ cup fat-free sour cream
1 tablespoon honey
1 tablespoon orange juice

Combine the fruits. Combine the sour cream, honey and orange juice. Pour over the mixed fruits. Toss to coat. Chill.

4 servings
0 fat grams per serving

English Pea Salad

2 boxes frozen English peas, thawed
1 medium onion, chopped
2 stalks celery, thinly sliced
4 ounces fat-free Cheddar cheese
1 tablespoon sweet pickle relish
commercial fat-free Ranch salad dressing

Combine all ingredients. Serve chilled.

6 servings
0 fat grams per serving

Fancy Fruit Salad

1 16-ounce can fruit cocktail, juice-packed, undrained
1 16-ounce can mandarin oranges, rinsed and drained
1 16-ounce can crushed pineapple, juice-packed,
   undrained
2 ripe bananas
1 .9-ounce box sugar-free vanilla instant pudding

Combine all ingredients. Chill.

0 fat grams per serving

Freezer Cole Slaw

1 medium cabbage, shredded
1 medium onion, chopped
1 green pepper, chopped
2 carrots, shredded
1 tablespoon salt
½ cup sugar
2 teaspoons dry mustard
2 cups cider vinegar

Combine the vegetables and the salt. Let stand 2 hours. Taste the vegetables. If they are too salty, rinse and drain. Combine the sugar, dry mustard and vinegar. Heat the dressing briefly and pour over the vegetables while still hot. Divide the slaw among pint freezer containers. Freeze. Thaw several hours before serving.

0 fat grams per serving

Fruit Salad with Poppy Seed Dressing

1 cup apple, chopped
1 cup seedless grapes
1 cup strawberries
1 cup melon balls, in season
2 bananas, sliced

Combine all of the fruits. Mix with poppy seed dressing. Serve chilled.

Dressing:
1 cup water
3 tablespoons cider vinegar
1 tablespoon cornstarch
3 tablespoons sugar
½ teaspoon dry mustard
2 teaspoons poppy seeds

Combine all of the ingredients and cook over medium heat until thickened. Let cool before mixing with the fruit.

6 servings
0 fat grams per serving

GELATIN SALADS

While these are usually considered salads, I actually use them as desserts, when I want something sweet. I usually keep a gelatin salad in my refrigerator at all times. Since the gelatin is a fat-free and sugar-free and other ingredients are fat-free, this is a guilt-free treat! I usually eat some several times a day. Just between you and me, I have been known to eat an entire recipe in one day. You can use your favorite sugar-free gelatin and favorite fruits to create your own gelatin treats.

Double Strawberry Delight

Prepare a large (.6-ounce) package of sugar-free strawberry gelatin, using the quick set method. When the gelatin is partially jelled, add 2 cups sliced strawberries (unsweetened) and ½ cup fat-free sour cream.

Chill in the refrigerator until jelled.

0 fat grams per serving

Lime Cooler

Prepare one large (.6-ounce) package of lime sugar-free gelatin according to the quick set method. When partially jelled, add 1 small can crushed pineapple (juice-pack), drained, and ½ cup fat-free cottage cheese. Chill until jelled.

0 fat grams per serving

German Potato Salad

6 medium potatoes, peeled and sliced
½ cup water
2 tablespoons all-purpose flour
4 tablespoons cider vinegar
¼ teaspoon celery seeds
2 tablespoons sugar or granulated sugar substitute
1 medium onion, thinly sliced
1 tablespoon imitation bacon bits

Boil the potatoes until tender. Meanwhile, combine the water and flour in a saucepan. Stir until the flour is dissolved. Add the vinegar and cook over medium heat until thickened. Add the celery seeds and sugar, or sugar substitute. Combine the potatoes and onion with the dressing. Serve warm, topped with the bacon bits.

6 servings
Less than 1 fat gram per serving

Guilt Free Potato Salad

6 baking potatoes, peeled, diced and cooked
2 stalks celery, chopped
1 medium onion, chopped
½ cup fat-free Ranch or Thousand Island dressing

Combine all ingredients. Serve chilled.

6 servings
0 fat grams per serving

Italian Vegetable and Pasta Salad

1 package frozen mixed broccoli, carrots and water
    chestnuts
8 ounces dry rotini, egg-free if possible, cooked
1 cup sliced mushrooms
1 medium onion, chopped
¾ cup bottled fat-free Italian dressing

Thaw the frozen vegetables under cold tap water. Drain completely. Add the remaining ingredients. Serve chilled.

4 servings
1 fat gram per serving

Marinated Cucumber and Onion Salad

1 large cucumber, very thinly sliced
1 large onion, very thinly sliced
⅓ cup cider vinegar
3 tablespoons sugar or granulated sugar substitute

Mix all ingredients. Chill, stirring occasionally.

4 servings
0 fat grams

Meal In One Dish Salad

8 cups shredded cabbage
½ pound cooked 98% fat-free ham, cut into thin strips
12 ounces fat-free shredded Cheddar cheese
1 medium onion, chopped
1 11-ounce can mandarin oranges, drained
fat-free Blue Cheese salad dressing

Toss all of the ingredients together in a large salad bowl.

4 servings
2 fat grams per serving

Middle Eastern Tabouli

1½ cups cooked bulgur
¼ cup lemon juice
¼ teaspoon garlic powder
2 tomatoes, diced
1 medium onion, chopped
1 tablespoon olive oil

Combine all of the ingredients except the tomatoes and the onions. Chill for several hours. Just before serving, add the vegetables.

4 servings
5 fat grams per serving

My Favorite Salad

I make this salad year round at mealtime and also as a snack. In the winter, when fresh tomatoes are not very good, I use cherry tomatoes or Italian plum tomatoes. Instead of croutons, I will sometimes crumble a few fat-free saltines over the top.

3 fresh tomatoes, chopped
1 medium onion, thinly sliced
1 large cucumber, thinly sliced
1 clove garlic, minced
4 ounces fat-free Cheddar cheese, shredded
commercial fat-free Italian dressing

Combine the vegetables and cheese. Top with the salad dressing.

4 servings
0 fat grams per serving

Spinach Salad

2 bags fresh spinach, torn into bite sized pieces
1 medium onion, thinly sliced
3 hard boiled egg whites, chopped
1 cup fat-free Cheddar cheese, shredded
1 tablespoon imitation bacon bits
commercial fat-free Ranch salad dressing

Combine all of the ingredients except the salad dressing. Add it immediately before serving.

6 servings
Less than 1 fat gram per serving

Springtime Salad

1 head iceberg lettuce, torn into bite-size pieces
1 cup fresh strawberries, sliced
1 mild onion, thinly sliced
1 cup fresh peaches or nectarines, peeled and sliced
commercial fat-free red French dressing

Combine the vegetables and fruits. Chill. Just before serving, add the salad dressing.

6 servings
0 fat grams per serving

Three Bean Salad

1 16-ounce can chickpeas, drained
1 16-ounce red kidney beans, drained
1 16-ounce can black beans, rinsed and drained
1 medium onion, chopped
1 green pepper, chopped
1 carrot, shredded
1 cup fat-free Italian salad dressing

Combine all of the above ingredients. Serve chilled.

4 servings
Less than 1 fat gram per serving

Turkey Salad

2 cups 99% fat-free, precooked turkey, chopped
1 cup celery, chopped
1 tablespoon mild onion, chopped
2 hard boiled egg whites, chopped
4 tablespoons fat-free Thousand Island or Ranch dress-
　　ing

Combine all ingredients. Serve chilled as a salad with tomato slices and fat-free crackers, or as a sandwich filling.

4 servings
2 fat grams per serving

Easy Blue Cheese Salad Dressing

There are a lot of excellent fat-free salad dressings on the
market, but sometimes it's fun to make them at home. This can
also be used as a dip with vegetables.

1 cup fat-free cottage cheese
½ cup skim milk
1 tablespoon crumbled blue cheese

Mix all ingredients. Chill

4 servings
1 fat gram per serving

Main Dishes

Make meatless main dishes and main dishes with just a bit of meat often. Pasta, grains, and vegetables should be the stars of a meal. Meat, if served, should only be a supporting player.

BEEF MAIN DISHES:

Baked Chow Mein

6 ounces browned ground round, drained and patted
    dry
3 cups cooked rice
1 onion chopped
2 stalks celery, finely chopped
1 cup mushrooms, sliced
1 16-ounce can mixed Chinese vegetables
1 10¾-ounce can 99% fat-free cream of mushroom soup

Combine all ingredients. Bake in a casserole dish for 30 minutes at 350°.

4 servings
5 fat grams per serving

Cheesy Ground Beef Casserole

This is one of those recipes that has been around for years. It has probably appeared at every pot luck supper ever held. It is very rich, full of ground beef, sour cream and cream cheese. It doesn't have to be that way. In a casserole, a little ground beef goes a long way, and our trusty fat-free sour cream, Cheddar cheese and cream cheese help lighten it up even more.

6 ounces browned ground round, rinsed and patted dry
¼ teaspoon garlic powder
1 16-ounce can tomato sauce
1 8-ounce package dry noodles, egg free if possible
1 medium onion chopped
8 ounces fat-free cream cheese, softened
8 ounces fat-free sour cream
4 ounces fat-free Cheddar cheese, shredded
no-stick cooking spray

Combine the ground round with the garlic and the tomato sauce. Prepare the noodles according to package directions. Combine the onion with the cream cheese, sour cream and Cheddar. Place a layer of the noodles in a baking dish that has been coated with no-stick cooking spray. Top with a layer of the meat sauce and then a layer of the cheese mixture. Repeat the layers. Bake at 350° for 30 minutes.

4 servings
5 fat grams per serving

Chili Mac

8 ounces ground top round or ultra-lean ground beef,
    browned and rinsed
1 medium onion, chopped
1 green pepper, chopped
½ teaspoon garlic powder
4 cups elbow macaroni, cooked
½ cup water
1 tablespoon chili powder
2 teaspoons ground cumin
1 16-ounce can Mexican style chunky tomato sauce
1 15 ounce can kidney beans, drained
1 6-ounce can tomato paste

Combine the cooked ground beef, onion and green pepper in a skillet. Cook until the vegetables are tender. Add the remaining ingredients and simmer 20 minutes, stirring occasionally.

4 servings
5 fat grams per serving

Corn Bread Pie

Filling:

1 onion, chopped
1 green pepper, chopped
no-stick cooking spray
6 ounces browned ground round, rinsed and patted dry
1 11-ounce can whole kernel corn, drained
1 tablespoon chili powder
1 16-ounce can chunky tomato sauce

Corn Bread Crust:

1 cup self-rising cornmeal mix
½ cup water
¼ cup fat-free egg substitute
2 tablespoons fat-free sour cream

Sauté the onion and green pepper in a skillet that has been coated with no-stick cooking spray. Add the remaining filling ingredients and place in a casserole dish. Prepare topping ingredients and pour over the filling. Bake at 350° for about 30 minutes, or until the topping is brown.

4 serving
0 fat grams per serving

English Cottage Pie
1 large onion, chopped
2 carrots, thinly sliced
1 cup frozen English peas
3 cups potatoes, peeled and diced
6 ounces browned ground round, rinsed and patted dry
1 can low-fat prepared brown gravy
1 tablespoon Worcestershire sauce
2 cups fat-free prepared mashed potatoes
butter-flavored cooking spray

Cook the onion, carrots, peas and diced potatoes in boiling water until tender. Combine with the beef, brown gravy and Worcestershire sauce. Pour into a casserole dish and spread the mashed potatoes over the top. Spray the potatoes with a bit of butter-flavored cooking spray. Bake at 375° for 30 minutes.

4 servings
5 fat grams per serving

Hamburger and Macaroni Casserole

6 ounces browned ground round, rinsed and patted dry
2 cups cooked macaroni
1 8-ounce can tomato sauce
1 16-ounce can tomatoes, chopped and drained
1 onion, diced
¼ teaspoon garlic powder
4 ounces fat-free sour cream

Combine the ground round, macaroni, tomato sauce, tomatoes, onion, garlic powder and sour cream. Pour into a casserole dish. Bake at 350° for 30 minutes.

4 servings
5 fat grams per serving

Hamburger Steak with Mushroom Gravy

1 pound ultra-lean ground beef or ground top round
1 10¾-ounce can 99% fat-free cream of mushroom soup
2 slices fat-free, reduced-calorie bread, made into
   crumbs
¼ cup fat-free egg substitute
½ medium onion, finely minced
¼ teaspoon garlic powder
⅛ teaspoon light salt
⅛ teaspoon black pepper
no-stick cooking spray
½ soup can water

Combine the ground beef, 2 tablespoons cream of mushroom soup, the bread crumbs, egg substitute, onion, garlic powder, salt and pepper. Thoroughly blend the ingredients. Shape into four small loaves. Place the loaves on a rack in a baking pan that has been coated with no-stick cooking spray. Bake at 350° for 20 minutes. Remove from the oven and place in a small baking dish that has been coated with no-stick cooking spray. Combine the remaining mushroom soup with ½ soup can of water. Pour over the meat. Return to the oven and bake 15 additional minutes.

4 servings
8 fat grams per serving

Inside Out Cabbage Rolls

Do you like cabbage rolls but don't have the time or inclination to go to all that trouble? You might try this recipe.

½ medium cabbage, chopped
1 medium onion, finely chopped
no-stick cooking spray
1 16-ounce can chunky tomato sauce
light salt and pepper to taste
6 ounces browned ground round, rinsed and patted dry
2 cups cooked rice

Sauté the cabbage and onion in a skillet that has been coated with no-stick cooking spray. When tender, combine with the remaining ingredients and pour into a casserole dish that has been sprayed with no-stick cooking spray. Bake at 350° for 20 minutes.

4 servings
4 fat grams per serving

Pepper Steak

12 ounces eye of round, all fat removed
no-stick cooking spray
1-ounce envelope dehydrated onion soup mix
2 cups water
2 medium green peppers, seeded and cut into strips
1 onion, cut into wedges
1½ tablespoons cornstarch
½ cup cold water

Slice the beef into thin strips. Stir-fry over medium heat until browned in a skillet or wok that has been coated with no-stick cooking spray. Add the dry soup mix and the water. Simmer, covered, for 15 minutes. Add the green pepper and onion. Simmer an additional 10 minutes. Mix the cornstarch with ½ cup cold water. Add to the skillet and stir. Continue to cook the mixture briefly, until thickened. Serve over cooked, hot rice.

4 servings
6 fat grams per serving

Pizzagetti

8 ounces angel hair pasta
1 16-ounce can fat-free pizza sauce or spaghetti sauce
no-stick cooking spray
6 ounces browned ground round, rinsed and patted dry
1 medium onion, thinly sliced
1 cup mushrooms, thinly sliced
1 green pepper, thinly sliced
4 ounces fat-free mozzarella cheese, shredded

Prepare the angel hair pasta according to package directions. When done, drain and mix with the pizza sauce. Place the pasta in a 9"x 13" baking dish that has been coated with no-stick cooking spray. Top the pasta with the beef, then with the vegetables. Bake uncovered at 350° for 20 minutes. While still very warm, just before serving, top with the cheese.

6 servings
3 fat grams per serving

Reduced Fat Meat Loaf
1 pound ultra-lean ground beef or ground top round
2 slices fat-free, reduced-calorie wheat bread, made into
   crumbs
½ medium onion, finely minced
½ green pepper, finely minced
1 carrot, shredded
¼ cup fat-free egg substitute
¼ teaspoon garlic powder
⅛ teaspoon light salt
⅛ teaspoon black pepper
4 tablespoons catsup, divided
no-stick cooking spray

Combine the beef, bread crumbs, vegetables, egg substitute, garlic powder, salt, pepper and 2 tablespoons catsup. Blend the ingredients thoroughly. Shape into four small individual loaves. Place the loaves on a rack in a baking pan that has been sprayed with no-stick cooking spray. Spread a bit of the remaining catsup atop each loaf. Bake at 350° for 20 minutes, or until done to your taste.

4 servings
7 fat grams per serving

Smothered Steak With Country Gravy

1 pound eye of round roast, trimmed of all fat and sliced
    into 4-ounce steaks
4 tablespoons all-purpose flour
½ teaspoon light salt
¼ teaspoon pepper
1 tablespoon vegetable oil
no-stick cooking spray
1½ cups water
8 ounces skim milk
4 teaspoons all-purpose flour

Place the steak slices between two pieces of plastic wrap and gently flatten with the flat side of a meat mallet. Combine the 4 tablespoons flour, ½ teaspoon salt and ¼ teaspoon pepper. Dredge the steak in the flour mixture. Coat the skillet with no-stick cooking spray. Brown the steaks over medium heat in the oil. Add the water and simmer, covered, for one hour. Check occasionally to see if more water is needed. Remove the meat from the pan and set aside. Combine the milk with the 4 teaspoons all-purpose flour. Add to the skillet. You may need to add additional water if much of it has cooked away. Stir the mixture until thickened. Return the meat to the gravy and simmer 5 minutes.

4 servings
11 fat grams per serving

Very Simple "Stroganoff"

6 ounces browned ground round, rinsed and patted dry
4 cups cooked rice
1 10¾-ounce can 99% fat-free cream of mushroom soup
1 cup fat-free sour cream
1 1-ounce package dehydrated onion soup mix
light salt and pepper to taste
no-stick cooking spray

Combine the ground round, rice, mushroom soup, sour cream, onion soup mix, salt and pepper. Pour into a casserole dish that has been coated with no-stick cooking spray. Bake for 30 minutes at 350°.

4 servings
5 fat grams per serving

CHICKEN MAIN DISHES

Barbecued Chicken

4 4-ounce chicken breast halves, skinned and boned
no-stick cooking spray
¾ cup water
¾ cup catsup
3 tablespoons cider vinegar
2 tablespoons granulated sugar substitute
1 teaspoon hickory smoke flavoring

Place the chicken breasts in a baking dish that has been sprayed with no-stick cooking spray. Combine the sauce ingredients and pour over the chicken. Bake, covered, for 30 minutes at 350°.

Shortcut: Use bottled barbecue sauce thinned with water. Read the label carefully. Some bottled sauces are rather high in fat, while some are fat-free.

4 servings
4 fat grams per serving

Chicken a la King

4 tablespoons all-purpose flour
1 ½-ounce package butter-flavored granules
2 cups skim milk
2 cups diced cooked chicken breast
3 hard boiled eggs, whites only, chopped
1 cup mushrooms, sliced and sautéed
1 tablespoon pimento, chopped

Prepare a white sauce using the flour, butter-flavored granules and milk. When thickened, add the remaining ingredients. Serve over cooked rice.

4 servings
4 fat grams per serving

Chicken Cacciatore
no-stick cooking spray
4 4-ounce chicken breast halves, boned and skinned
1 medium onion, sliced
1 pound fresh mushrooms, sliced
1 bell pepper, sliced
1 15-ounce can tomato sauce
1 15-ounce can tomatoes, chopped and drained
1-2 teaspoons dried oregano, to taste
¼ teaspoon garlic powder

Coat a skillet with no-stick cooking spray. Sauté the chicken over medium heat until cooked throughout and lightly browned on both sides. Remove the chicken from the skillet. Sauté the onion, mushrooms and peppers until tender-crisp. Add the tomato sauce, the tomatoes, the oregano and the garlic to the vegetables in the skillet. Return the chicken to the skillet. Simmer a few minutes to blend the flavors. Good with pasta or rice.

4 servings
4 fat grams per serving

Chicken-Mushroom Casserole

4 4-ounce boneless, skinless chicken breast halves, cooked and
 chopped or 3 5-ounce cans chunk white chicken packed in
 water.
1 10¾-ounce can 99% fat-free cream of mushroom soup
8 ounces fat-free sour cream
1 package long grain and wild rice mix, prepared
 according to package directions, omitting margarine
 or butter
1 8-ounce can sliced water chestnuts, drained
1 4-ounce can sliced mushrooms, drained
1 medium onion, chopped
2 stalks celery, chopped
no-stick cook spray

Mix the cooked chicken cubes with the mushroom soup and
the sour cream. Add the cooked rice, water chestnuts, mushrooms, onion and celery. Turn into a 2-quart casserole dish that
has been sprayed with no-stick cooking spray. Bake at 350°, covered, for 30 minutes.

4 servings
6 fat grams per serving

Chicken Casserole

1 8-ounce package angel hair pasta
2 cups cooked chicken breast meat, cubed
1 10 ¾-ounce can 99% fat-free cream of chicken soup
1 cup fat-free sour cream
1 cup sliced mushrooms
light salt and pepper to taste
no-stick cooking spray

Cook the pasta according to package directions. Drain well. Add the chicken, soup, sour cream, mushrooms, salt and pepper. Pour into a casserole dish that has been coated with no-stick cooking spray. Bake at 375° for 20 minutes.

4 servings
5 fat grams per serving

Crispy Broiled Chicken

6 4-ounce chicken breast halves, skinned and boned
no-stick cooking spray
2 tablespoons cornmeal
2 cloves garlic, minced, or ¼ teaspoon garlic powder
½ teaspoon black pepper
3 tablespoons lemon juice
2 teaspoons vegetable oil

Place the chicken breasts in a 9" x 13" baking dish that has been coated with cooking spray. Combine cornmeal, garlic, pepper, lemon juice and oil. Spread the cornmeal mixture on top of each breast. Refrigerate for one hour. Broil 8" from heat until chicken is done and topping is crispy.

6 servings
7 fat grams per serving

The Easiest Chicken and Dumplings Ever

4 4-ounce chicken breasts halves, skinned and boned
6 cups water
1 13.5-ounce package fat-free flour tortillas
1 10¾-ounce can 99% fat-free cream of chicken soup
½ cup water

Cover the chicken with water and boil until tender. Remove the chicken from the broth and cut into bite-size pieces. Set aside. Cut the tortillas into approximately 2" square pieces. Bring the chicken broth to a boil and drop in the tortilla pieces, one at a time, stirring frequently to keep the tortillas from sticking together. They will be done in a short time. Combine the cream of chicken soup with ½ cup water. Add to the dumplings. Return the chicken pieces to the pot. Good with English peas and sliced tomatoes.

6 servings
4 fat grams per serving.

Easy Italian Chicken

6 4-ounce chicken breast halves, skinned and boned
1 cup fat-free Italian salad dressing
olive oil-flavored no-stick cooking spray

Marinate the chicken breasts in the salad dressing for at least 20 minutes. Remove the chicken from the marinade. Place in a baking dish that has been sprayed with olive oil-flavored no-stick cooking spray. Also spray the chicken with the cooking spray. Bake at 375° for 25 minutes.

6 servings
4 fat grams per serving

Greek Chicken

A personal favorite. Very easy to fix and very good served with cooked rice.

4 4-ounce skinned and boned chicken breast halves
¼ cup lemon juice
1 clove garlic, minced or ⅛ teaspoon garlic powder
1 teaspoon dried oregano
½ teaspoon coarsely ground black pepper
butter-flavored no-stick cooking spray

Sprinkle the chicken breasts with the lemon juice, then the garlic, oregano and pepper. Let marinate 10 minutes. Place the breasts in a baking dish that has been coated with the butter-flavored cooking spray. Lightly coat the breasts with the cooking spray. Bake at 350°, 15-20 minutes until well done and lightly browned. Do not overcook.

4 servings
4 fat grams per serving

Lemon Chicken

4 4-ounce chicken breast halves, skinned and boned
¼ cup lemon juice
1 teaspoon dried tarragon
¼ teaspoon garlic powder

Place each chicken breast on a 12" square of aluminum foil. Sprinkle 1 tablespoon lemon juice on each breast, then sprinkle with the tarragon and garlic powder. Carefully fold the foil so that the lemon juice can't run out. Bake at 350° for 20-25 minutes.

4 servings
4 fat grams per serving

Moist and Tender Oven Fried Chicken

4 4-ounce chicken breast halves, boned and skinned
1 cup cold buttermilk
¾ cup fine, dry bread crumbs
1 teaspoon garlic powder
1 teaspoon dried oregano
1 tablespoon grated Parmesan cheese
⅛ teaspoon light salt
no-stick cooking spray

Place the chicken in the buttermilk, making sure that the buttermilk coats each chicken piece. Place in the refrigerator for 4 hours. Meanwhile, combine the crumbs, garlic powder, oregano, Parmesan cheese and salt. Remove the chicken from the buttermilk and roll each piece in the crumb mixture. Place the chicken into a baking pan that has been sprayed with no-stick cooking spray. Bake at 425° for 25 minutes, turning halfway through the cooking time.

4 servings
4 fat grams per serving

Mongolian Chicken

Mongolian beef is a very popular Chinese restaurant entrée that my family loves for me to make at home. While it can be prepared with a fairly low-fat cut of beef, such as eye of round, it is equally good with chicken breast or, for even less fat, turkey breast.

4 4-ounce chicken breast halves, boned and skinned
2 tablespoons fat-free chicken broth
2 bunches green onions, including tops, cut into 2"
    pieces
1 tablespoon brown sugar
½ teaspoon sesame oil
3 tablespoons reduced-sodium soy sauce
1 tablespoon dark soy sauce
1 dried red pepper or dried red pepper flakes to taste

Cut the chicken breasts into bite size pieces. Bring the chicken broth to a boil over high heat in a wok or skillet. Sauté the chicken in the broth. Set aside. Sauté the green onions in the same manner. Mix the remaining ingredients together and add to the wok or skillet, along with the chicken. Serve with hot, cooked rice.

4 servings
5 fat grams per serving

No Watch Chicken Dinner

4 4-ounce breast halves, skinned and boned
1 tablespoon Dijon mustard
¼ teaspoon garlic powder
1 teaspoon tarragon
1 teaspoon paprika
4 yellow squash, sliced
1 large onion, sliced
3 baking potatoes, sliced

Place each chicken breast on a 12" square piece of foil. Top with a bit of Dijon mustard and a sprinkle of the garlic powder and tarragon and paprika. Add sliced squash, onion and potatoes. Tightly close the foil packets and place in a shallow baking dish. Bake at 400° for 30 minutes.

4 servings
4 fat grams per serving

Oniony Oven Fried Chicken

½ cup fine, dry bread crumbs
1 1-ounce package dehydrated onion soup mix
4 4-ounce chicken breast halves, skinned and boned
no-stick cooking spray

Combine the dry ingredients. Spray the chicken very lightly with the cooking spray. Coat each piece of chicken with the dry mixture. Spray the coated pieces again. Bake at 350° for 20-25 minutes.

4 servings
5 fat grams per serving

Oven Fried Sesame Chicken

While sesame seeds are quite high in fat, they add so much to a dish that a few shouldn't hurt from time to time. A tablespoon contains 4.5 fat grams, but they are so small that just a few go a long way.

2 tablespoons sesame seeds
4 tablespoons fine, dry bread crumbs
¼ teaspoon pepper
4 4-ounce chicken breast halves, boned and skinned
2 tablespoons soy sauce
no-stick cooking spray

Combine sesame seeds, bread crumbs and pepper. Dip chicken breasts in the soy sauce and roll in the sesame seed mixture. Place the chicken on a baking sheet that has been coated with no-stick cooking spray. Also spray each breast after placing them on the baking sheet. Bake for 25 minutes at 450° or until browned. Turn halfway through cooking time. Do not overcook.

4 servings
7 fat grams per serving

Pan Fried Chicken Breasts

4 4-ounce chicken breast halves, boneless and skinless
1 cup fine, dry bread crumbs
½ teaspoon garlic powder
⅛ teaspoon light salt
no-stick cooking spray
1 tablespoon canola oil

Lightly flatten the chicken breasts. Combine the crumbs, garlic powder and salt. Dredge the chicken in the crumb mixture. Set aside for a few minutes to help the coating adhere to the chicken when cooked. Spray a skillet with no-stick cooking spray. Place the pan over medium heat. When it is hot, add one half of the oil, swirling the pan to evenly coat the bottom. Add the chicken. Pan fry the chicken till brown on one side. Add the remaining oil and turn the chicken to cook the other side until brown.

4 servings
9 fat grams per serving

Stir-Fried Chicken and Vegetables

4 4-ounce chicken breast halves, skinned and boned, cut
    into strips
no-stick cooking spray
1 large onion, sliced
1 green pepper, sliced
2 tablespoons cornstarch
3 tablespoons soy sauce
1 cup fat-free chicken broth
2 large tomatoes, cut into wedges

Stir-fry the chicken in a skillet or wok that has been coated with no-stick cooking spray. Remove from the skillet or wok and stir-fry the onion and pepper in the same manner. Combine the sauce ingredients. Add to the skillet, along with the chicken. When sauce is thickened, add the tomatoes. Continue cooking until tomatoes are heated through. Serve with rice.

4 servings
4 fat grams per serving

Sweet and Sour Chicken

4 4-ounce chicken breast halves, skinned and boned, cut into
    strips
 no-stick cooking spray
1 8-ounce can pineapple tidbits, juice-packed, juice
    reserved
1 8-ounce can water chestnuts, sliced
1 carrot, thinly sliced
1 green pepper, cut into cubes

Sauce:
½ cup tomato paste
½ cup water
½ cup reserved pineapple juice
3 tablespoons brown sugar or granulated brown sugar
    substitute
3 tablespoons vinegar

Stir-fry the chicken in a skillet or wok that has been coated with no-stick cooking spray. Remove. Stir-fry the pineapple and vegetables in the same way. Combine the sauce ingredients and add to the vegetables, along with the chicken. Stir until thickened. Serve with rice.

4 servings
4 fat grams per serving

Teriyaki Kabobs

1 8-ounce can pineapple chunks, juice reserved
½ cup light soy sauce
¼ cup sherry
1 tablespoon sugar
½ teaspoon ground ginger
¼ teaspoon garlic powder
4 4-ounce chicken breasts, boned and skinned, each cut
    into 4 pieces
1 teaspoon cornstarch
16 cherry tomatoes
16 mushrooms

Combine the reserved pineapple juice, soy sauce, sherry, sugar, ground ginger and garlic powder. Add the chicken and marinate 20 minutes. Remove the chicken from the marinade and set aside. Add the cornstarch to the marinade and boil until slightly thickened.

Thread 4 pieces of chicken breast, 4 pineapple chunks, 4 cherry tomatoes and 4 mushrooms onto each of 4 skewers. Grill over hot coals until done, brushing with the marinade frequently.

4 servings
4 fat grams per serving

FISH MAIN DISHES

Always Moist Fish in Foil
For each serving:
4-ounce fish fillet
no-stick cooking spray
dash of dill or tarragon to taste

Place the fish fillet on a square of aluminum foil that has been sprayed with no-stick cooking spray. Coat the fillet with a bit of the cooking spray. Sprinkle with herbs as desired. Tightly close the foil. Close carefully so that juices cannot leak out during cooking. Place the foil packets in a baking dish. Bake at 400° for 15 minutes per inch of thickness.

1 serving
Less than 2 fat grams per serving

Baked Flounder
1 pound flounder fillets
1 10¾ ounce can 99% fat-free cream of mushroom
    soup
1 4-ounce can sliced mushrooms
chopped fresh parsley
no-stick cooking spray

Place the fish in a baking dish that has been coated with no-stick cooking spray. Cover with the undiluted soup. Top with the mushrooms. Sprinkle with chopped parsley. Bake at 400° for 30 minutes

4 servings
3 fat grams per serving

Baked Tuna Croquettes
1 7-ounce can water packed tuna
2 slices fat-free, reduced-calorie bread, made into
    crumbs
2 tablespoons onion, chopped
¼ cup fat-free sour cream
1 teaspoon lemon juice
2 tablespoons evaporated skim milk
¼ cup wheat germ
no-stick cooking spray

Combine the tuna, bread crumbs, onion, sour cream, lemon juice and evaporated skim milk. Shape the combined mixture into croquettes. Roll in the wheat germ. Place on a baking sheet that has been coated with no-stick cooking spray. Also spray the croquettes lightly with the cooking spray. Bake at 375° for 20 minutes.

4 servings
3 fat grams per serving

Dilled Baked Fish
2 pounds fish fillets
butter-flavored no-stick cooking spray
2 teaspoons chopped parsley
1 teaspoon dill weed

Spray a baking dish with butter-flavored no-stick cooking spray. Arrange fish fillets in the dish, then spray the fillets with the butter-flavored spray. Sprinkle with the parsley and the dill weed. Cover tightly with foil. Bake at 400° for 30 minutes.

8 servings
2 fat grams per serving

Gulf Coast Broiled Fish
1 pound fish fillets
no-stick cooking spray
4 teaspoons reduced-fat mayonnaise
lemon pepper, to taste
garlic powder, to taste

Place the fish in a baking dish that has been coated with no-stick cooking spray. Spread 1 teaspoon reduced-fat mayonnaise on each piece. Sprinkle with lemon pepper and garlic powder. Broil 4" from the heat source until done.

4 servings
3 fat grams per serving

Oven Fried Fish
This recipe can also be used with skinless, boneless chicken breasts.

⅓ cup fine, dry bread crumbs
⅛ teaspoon light salt
⅛ teaspoon pepper
1 tablespoon vegetable oil
4 4-ounce fish fillets
no-stick cooking spray

Combine the crumbs, salt, pepper and oil in a small bowl. Blend the mixture thoroughly. Sprinkle the tops of the fish fillets with the crumb mixture. Place the fillets in a baking dish that has been coated with no-stick cooking spray. Bake at 450° until the fish is opaque and flakes easily.

4 servings
5 fat grams per serving

Shrimp Creole

1 pound medium shrimp, peeled and deveined
no-stick cooking spray
1 clove garlic, minced or ⅛ teaspoon garlic powder
1 medium onion, chopped
1 green pepper, chopped
3 tablespoons all-purpose flour
1 cup water
1 8-ounce can tomato sauce
½ teaspoon red pepper
light salt and pepper to taste

Sauté the shrimp in a saucepan that has been coated with no-stick cooking spray. Remove. Sauté the vegetables in the same manner. Add the flour to the water. Add to the vegetable mixture. Add the tomato sauce and the seasoning, as well as the shrimp. Simmer for about 20 minutes. Serve with rice.

4 servings
2 fat grams per serving

Shrimp Scampi

1 tablespoon vegetable oil
2 tablespoons fresh lemon juice
¼ teaspoon garlic powder
dash of hot sauce, or to taste
butter-flavored no-stick cooking spray
1 pound medium fresh shrimp, peeled and deveined

Combine the oil, lemon juice, garlic powder and hot sauce in a skillet that has been coated with butter-flavored no-stick cooking spray. Sauté the shrimp in the oil mixture until they turn pink. Serve with rice.

4 servings
6 fat grams per serving

Tuna Casserole-Again?

The title of this recipe refers to the fact that every cook in America has probably heard those words. This dish is a reliable old standby that we have all probably served too much, but it is good, quick and easy.

1 10¾-ounce can 99% fat-free cream of mushroom
    soup
½ cup fat-free sour cream
¾ cup skim milk
7-ounce can white tuna, packed in water
2 cups cooked medium noodles
1 cup sliced mushrooms
light salt and pepper to taste
no-stick cooking spray

Combine the soup, sour cream and milk. Add tuna, noodles, mushrooms, salt and pepper. Pour the tuna mixture into a casserole dish that has been coated with the cooking spray. Bake at 350° for 30 minutes.

4 servings
2 fat grams per serving

Tuna Puff

1 7-ounce can white tuna, packed in water
½ cup chopped onion
2½ cups fat-free prepared mashed potatoes
¼ cup fat-free egg substitute
4 ounces fat-free Cheddar cheese, shredded
light salt and pepper to taste
no-stick cooking spray

Combine the tuna, onion, mashed potatoes, egg substitute, cheese, salt and pepper. Pour into a baking dish that has been coated with no-stick cooking spray. Bake at 350° for 30 minutes.

4 servings
1 fat gram per serving

HAM MAIN DISHES

Barbecued Ham and Corn Casserole
8 ounces 98% fat-free precooked ham
1 medium onion, chopped
1 medium green pepper, chopped
1 16-ounce can whole kernel corn, drained
1 cup catsup
1 teaspoon chili powder
¼ teaspoon garlic powder
dash of hot sauce

Sauté the vegetables and ham in a skillet that has been coated with no-stick cooking spray. Add the other ingredients. Pour into a casserole dish and bake 20 minutes at 350°.

4 servings
2 fat grams per serving

Calico Beans

½ pound 98% fat-free cooked ham, diced
1 chopped onion
½ cup catsup
2 teaspoons mustard
1 tablespoon vinegar
2 tablespoons brown sugar or 2 tablespoons granulated
    brown sugar substitute
1 16-ounce can fat-free baked beans
1 16-ounce can kidney beans, drained
1 19-ounce can chickpeas, drained
no-stick cooking spray

Combine all of the ingredients and pour into a casserole dish that has been coated with no-stick cooking spray. Bake at 350°, uncovered, for 40 minutes.

6 servings
2 fat grams per serving

Chunky Ham Casserole

6 ounces 98% fat-free precooked ham, chopped
1 8-ounce package noodles, cooked according to pack-
    age directions
1 10¾-ounce can 99% fat-free cream of mushroom soup
½ cup fat-free sour cream
1 teaspoon poppy seeds
1 tablespoon dehydrated onion flakes

Combine all of the ingredients and pour into a casserole dish. Bake at 350° for 20 minutes

4 servings
4 fat grams per serving

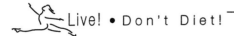

Creamy Ham and Macaroni Casserole

1 green pepper, chopped
1 medium onion, chopped
no-stick cooking spray
3 tablespoons all-purpose flour
1½ cups skim milk
light salt and pepper to taste
1 8-ounce package macaroni, egg free if possible,
    cooked
8 ounces 98% fat-free cooked ham, cut into cubes
1 cup fat-free cottage cheese

Sauté the vegetables in a skillet that has been sprayed with no-stick cooking spray. Stir in the flour, then the milk, salt and pepper. Bring to a boil, stirring constantly. Add the macaroni, ham and cottage cheese. Pour into a casserole dish and bake at 350° for 30 minutes.

4 servings
3 fat grams per serving

Ham and Cheese Crepes

Versatile crepes can be lifesavers when unexpected company comes for dinner. Keep a supply of unfilled crepes in the freezer. Then just prepare a quick filling and you're ready to eat.

8 crepes (see recipe index)
1 cup fat-free cottage cheese
6 ounces 98% fat-free precooked ham, cut into match-
    stick sized pieces
4 ounces fat-free Cheddar cheese, shredded
1 10¾-ounce can 99% fat-free cream of mushroom soup
½ soup can water or skim milk
1 4-ounce can sliced mushrooms, drained

Combine the cottage cheese, ham and Cheddar cheese. Place several tablespoons of filling down the center of each crepe, then fold the sides over the filling. Place the filled crepes in a 9" x 13" baking dish. Combine the mushroom soup, water or milk and sliced mushrooms. Pour over the crepes. Bake for 20 minutes at 350°.

4 servings
8 fat grams per serving

Ham With Raisin Sauce

Ham with raisin sauce is a popular Sunday dinner entrée that you can serve while staying well within your fat gram goal. Many of the boneless, precooked hams in the grocery store today are 98%-99% fat-free and have only 100 calories and 3 fat grams per 3-ounce serving.

1 99% fat-free precooked ham
¼ cup seedless raisins
½ cup water
½ cup brown sugar or substitute to equal ½ cup sugar
2 teaspoons cornstarch
¼ teaspoon light salt
1 teaspoon vinegar

Wrap the ham in foil and bake at 350° for approximately 1 hour. Meanwhile, simmer the raisins in the water for 10 minutes. Mix the remaining ingredients and add to the raisin-water mixture. Simmer 3 minutes or until thickened.

3 fat grams per 3 ounce serving of ham
0 fat grams for the sauce

Microwave Ham Loaves

½ cup fat-free egg substitute
2 slices fat-free, reduced-calorie bread, made into
     crumbs
¼ cup finely chopped onion
2 teaspoons Dijon mustard
2 5-ounce cans chunk ham or 10 ounces ground 98%
     fat-free cooked ham
3 tablespoons reduced-sugar orange marmalade

Combine the egg substitute, bread crumbs, onion, mustard and ham. Shape into 4 individual loaves. Place in a microwave safe dish with a cover. Microwave on high for 6 minutes, rotating after 3 minutes. Spread each loaf with marmalade and microwave uncovered for 1 minute.

4 servings
7 fat grams each serving

Skillet Cabbage and Ham

½ pound 98% fat-free cooked ham, chopped
no-stick cooking spray
½ head cabbage, coarsely chopped
1 onion, chopped
¼ cup water

Briefly sauté the cooked ham in a skillet that has been sprayed with no-stick cooking spray. Add the cabbage, onion and water. Cook, covered, over medium heat, for 15 minutes or until the cabbage is done to your preference.

4 servings
2 fat grams per serving

TURKEY MAIN DISHES

Almost Instant Turkey and Dressing
You can prepare this when you have the taste but not the time for the holiday favorite.

1 onion chopped
½ cups celery chopped
no-stick cooking spray
1 box corn bread stuffing mix
1 16-ounce can fat-free chicken broth
¼ cup fat-free egg substitute
8 1-ounce slices 99% fat-free precooked turkey
1 10¼ -ounce can low-fat prepared turkey or chicken
    gravy

Sauté the onion and celery in a skillet that has been sprayed with no-stick cooking spray. Prepare the boxed stuffing mix according to package directions, omitting the margarine. Use the chicken broth instead of the water specified in the directions. Add the sautéed vegetables and the egg substitute to the dressing. Pour into a casserole dish and bake at 350° for 30 minutes or until brown. Serve with the heated, sliced turkey and gravy.

4 servings
4 fat grams per serving

Chinese Lo-Mein

Another staple around our house. Adding lots of vegetables and a little meat to the pasta makes this a one dish meal.

8 ounces angel hair pasta, egg free if possible
8 ounces precooked 99% fat-free turkey breast, cut into
    matchstick size pieces
1 cup cabbage, shredded
1 cup fresh mushrooms, sliced
1 onion, cut into wedges
no-stick cooking spray
light soy sauce to taste

Cook the pasta according to package directions. Drain well. Sauté the turkey, cabbage, mushrooms and onion in a skillet that has been coated with no-stick cooking spray. When the vegetables are tender-crisp, add the mixture to the cooked pasta. Toss with the light soy sauce before serving.

4 servings
3 fat grams per serving

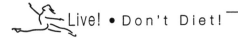

Turkey Cutlets, Scallopini
4 4-ounce fresh turkey breast cutlets
butter-flavored no-stick cooking spray
1 cup mushrooms, sliced
⅛ teaspoon garlic powder
1 teaspoon dried rosemary
fresh lemon juice

Sauté the turkey cutlets in a skillet that has been sprayed with butter-flavored no-stick cooking spray. Remove the cooked turkey. Sauté the mushrooms in the same manner. Return the turkey to the skillet and sprinkle with the garlic and rosemary, as well as a bit of fresh lemon juice. Serve with rice or noodles.

4 servings
4 fat grams per serving

WEINER MAIN DISHES

Hot Dog Casserole
This casserole is a lot like hot dogs without the bun. Great with mashed potatoes.

1 cup catsup
¼ cup prepared mustard
sugar substitute to equal ¼ cup sugar
2 tablespoons Worcestershire sauce
2 16-ounce cans baked beans, drained
1 medium onion, chopped
1 green pepper, chopped
no-stick cooking spray
1 pound 97% fat-free wieners
1 16-ounce can sauerkraut

Mix the catsup, mustard, sugar substitute and Worcestershire together. Set aside. Pour the baked beans into a baking dish that has been coated with no-stick cooking spray. Sauté the onion and pepper in a skillet that has been coated with cooking spray. Spread the onion and pepper over the beans. Spread half of the sauce over the onion and pepper. Place the wieners on top of the sauce. Top with the sauerkraut and then the remaining sauce. Bake at 350° for 25-30 minutes.

5 servings
2 fat grams per serving

Weiners and Baked Beans

This is an old standby for grocery shopping night. After working all day, then buying groceries and putting them up, I really am in a hurry to get out of the kitchen. This is super quick and popular with the family too.

2 16-ounce cans fat-free baked beans
no-stick cooking spray
1 chopped onion
5 97% fat-free weiners, cut into thirds

Pour the baked beans into a 2 quart casserole that has been sprayed with no-stick cooking spray. Add the chopped onion and mix well. Top with the weiners. Bake uncovered at 350° until the weiners are lightly browned and the beans are bubbly. Good with Mom's Mashed Potatoes or in a real pinch, instant mashed potatoes.

4 servings
Less than 2 fat grams per serving

MEATLESS MAIN DISHES

Cheese Enchiladas
12 corn tortillas (1 8-ounce package)
2 cups fat-free cottage cheese
4 ounces fat-free Cheddar cheese
1 medium onion, finely minced
1 15-ounce can Mexican style tomato sauce

Briefly warm the tortillas to make them pliable. If you have a microwave oven, you can just make a few slits in the package and heat them on high for about 30 seconds. Combine the cheeses and the onion. Place a spoonful of the cheese filling on each tortilla and roll up. Place the enchiladas in a 9" x 13" casserole after lightly coating the bottom of the dish with tomato sauce. Pour the remaining sauce over the enchiladas. Cover tightly with foil and bake at 350° for 30 minutes.

4 servings
3 fat grams per serving

Lasagna

1 26¾-ounce can fat-free spaghetti sauce
9 lasagna noodles, cooked
2 cups fat-free cottage cheese
¼ cup fine, dry bread crumbs
1 cup fat-free shredded mozzarella cheese
1 tablespoon grated Parmesan cheese
1 teaspoon oregano
¼ teaspoon garlic powder, or 2 cloves garlic, minced

Place a thin layer of spaghetti sauce in a 8" x 11½" baking dish. Place three cooked lasagna noodles on top of the sauce. Combine the cottage cheese, bread crumbs mozzarella cheese, Parmesan cheese, oregano and garlic. Place one half of the cheese mixture on the noodles. Top the cheese layer with one third of the remaining spaghetti sauce. Repeat the layers until all ingredients are used. Bake at 350° for 30 minutes. Let stand for 15 minutes before serving.

8 servings
1 fat gram per serving

Manicotti Florentine

2 cups fat-free cottage cheese
½ cup fat-free mozzarella cheese, shredded
1 tablespoon grated Parmesan cheese
¼ cup fine, dry bread crumbs
1 10-ounce package frozen chopped spinach, thawed and
    squeezed dry
¼ teaspoon garlic powder
1 teaspoon dried oregano
12 manicotti shells, cooked
1 26¾-ounce can fat-free spaghetti sauce

Combine the cottage cheese, mozzarella, Parmesan, dry bread crumbs, spinach, garlic and oregano. Stuff each shell with some of the cheese mixture. Spread a thin layer of spaghetti sauce in the bottom of a 9" x 13" baking dish. Place the filled shells in the dish. Cover with the remaining spaghetti sauce. Cover tightly with aluminum foil and bake at 350° for 30 minutes. Uncover and let stand 15 minutes before serving.

4 servings
2 fat grams per serving

Mexican Lasagna
no-stick cooking spray
1 8-ounce bottle taco sauce
1 8-ounce package corn tortillas
2 16-ounce cans fat-free refried beans
2 cups fat-free cottage cheese
1 green pepper minced
1 onion, minced
4 ounces fat-free Cheddar cheese, shredded

Spray a 9" x 13" baking dish with no-stick cooking spray. Spread a thin layer of taco sauce in the pan. Place a single layer of tortillas on the sauce. Spread the contents of one can of refried beans on the tortillas, followed by 1 cup of cottage cheese. Add ½ of the pepper and onion, then ½ of the Cheddar cheese. Dollop spoonfuls of taco sauce evenly on top. Repeat all the layers. Cover with foil and bake at 350° for 30 minutes.

6 large servings
3 fat grams per serving

No Bake Lasagna Style Casserole

I make this dish once a week. It is one of my favorites because it is so much fun to see a huge plateful and to know that I can eat it all without guilt! I usually serve it with sliced tomatoes, onions and cucumbers marinated in Italian dressing and garlic bread.

12-ounce package rotini or pasta shells, egg free if possible
1 cup fresh mushrooms, sliced
1 medium onion, chopped
1 medium green pepper, chopped
1 cup fat-free cottage cheese
¼ teaspoon garlic powder
1 teaspoon oregano
½ of a 26¾-ounce can fat-free spaghetti sauce, heated

Cook the pasta according to package directions. When done, drain thoroughly. Add the vegetables to the hot pasta in the cooking vessel. Allow the pasta and vegetables to stand, covered, for about 5 minutes to allow the heat of the pasta to lightly steam the vegetables. Add the cottage cheese, garlic powder and oregano to the pasta just before serving. Place each serving on a dinner plate and top with heated sauce.

4 servings
Less than 2 fat grams per serving

Spaghetti Dinner

I used to spend half a day making spaghetti sauce. Now I open a can. My husband likes it even better than my homemade sauce. I usually purchase the basic sauce and dress it up by adding some additional vegetables.

1 26¾-ounce can fat-free spaghetti sauce
1 cup sliced mushrooms
1 medium onion, chopped

Combine all ingredients and simmer until the vegetables are tender. Serve over cooked spaghetti. Good with salad and garlic bread.

4-6 servings
0 fat grams per serving

Vegetable Lasagna

1 medium eggplant, peeled and sliced
3 cups zucchini, sliced
no-stick cooking spray
2 cups fat-free cottage cheese
¼ cup fine, dry breadcrumbs
½ cup fat-free mozzarella, shredded
1 tablespoon Parmesan cheese, grated
1 26¾-ounce can fat-free spaghetti sauce

Sauté the eggplant slices, then the zucchini slices, in a skillet that has been sprayed with no-stick cooking spray. Place half of the cooked vegetables in a single layer in an 8" x 11½" casserole dish. Mix the cottage cheese with the breadcrumbs, the mozzarella and 2 teaspoons of the Parmesan cheese. Top the vegetables with ½ of the cheese mixture, then half of the spaghetti sauce. Repeat the layers. Bake at 350° for 20-25 minutes, uncovered. Let stand 10 minutes before serving. Just before serving, sprinkle with the remaining Parmesan cheese.

6 servings
Less than 1 fat gram per serving

VEGETABLES

Vegetables should be the heart and soul of low-fat meals. Buy and enjoy a wide variety of vegetables and prepare them in an interesting manner. Herbs, spices, butter-flavored granules, lemon juice, garlic, and homemade or commercially prepared gravies or sauces can add punch to plain vegetables. Even plain ketchup is not bad in a pinch. You can also add a can of 99% fat-free cream soup, a little fat-free sour cream, and fat-free shredded or sliced Cheddar cheese to vegetables to create an easy, cheesy casserole. It's a good idea to keep a lot of aromatic vegetables, such as onion, sweet peppers and celery on hand. They can be chopped and included in any number of dishes to add bulk and flavor. You can even keep a supply of chopped aromatic vegetables in the freezer. Just add a handful to any dish if it strikes your fancy.

Busy Day Pinto Beans
2 cans pinto beans, rinsed and drained
½ cup chopped green pepper
½ cup chopped onion
½ cup catsup
1 tablespoon Worcestershire sauce

Combine all of the ingredients in a saucepan. Cook over medium heat until the onions and peppers are tender.

4 servings
Less than 1 fat gram per serving

Country Style Black-Eyed Peas
1 cup dried black-eyed peas
6 cups hot water
3 chicken bouillon cubes
1 onion, chopped
1 whole hot pepper

After washing the peas, combine them in a saucepan with the rest of the ingredients. Simmer over low heat for 2-2½ hours or until tender. Discard the pepper before serving.

4 servings
Less than 1 fat gram per serving

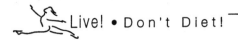

Deluxe Refried Beans

Serve these as an accompaniment to any Mexican style meal, or as a dip with baked tortilla chips.

2 16-ounce cans fat-free refried beans
1 medium onion, finely chopped
4 ounces fat-free Cheddar cheese
1 4-ounce can chopped chili peppers
no-stick cooking spray
fat-free sour cream

Mix the beans, onion, cheese and chili peppers. Pour into a casserole dish that has been coated with no-stick cooking spray. Bake at 350° until bubbly. When serving, add a dollop of sour cream to individual portions.

4 large servings
Less than 2 fat grams per serving

English Pea Casserole

This old standby is still popular with my family. Many food critics disdain the use of mushroom soup in recipes. I make no apologies for using it frequently. It adds a creamy richness to dishes, and thankfully is available in an almost fat-free version.

2 16-ounce cans small English peas, drained
1 10¾-ounce can 99% fat-free cream of mushroom soup
3 tablespoons fat-free sour cream
2 tablespoons dehydrated minced onion
1 8-ounce can sliced water chestnuts, drained
4 ¾-ounce slices fat-free Swiss or Cheddar cheese
1 slice fat-free, reduced-calorie bread, made into crumbs

Combine the peas, mushroom soup, sour cream, onion and water chestnuts. Pour half of the mixture into a 1½ quart casserole dish. Top with the cheese slices. Pour the remaining mixture over the cheese slices. Top the casserole with the bread crumbs. Bake at 350° for 20 minutes, or until the crumbs are brown.

Variation: Use 2 16-ounce cans of asparagus or mixed vegetables.

6 servings
Less than 2 fat grams per serving

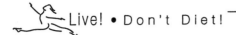

Green Beans and Potatoes

2 16-ounce cans green beans, rinsed and drained
8 new potatoes, quartered
1 cup water
1 chicken bouillon cube

Combine all of the ingredients in a saucepan. Simmer, covered, over medium heat until the potatoes are tender.

4 servings
0 fat grams per serving

Hopping John

Hopping John is a traditional southern dish. It is often served on New Year's Day to bring good luck in the coming year. Because it contains both blackeyed peas and rice, it is especially filling. Since part of the good luck is supposed to come from cooking the peas, it is usually prepared from scratch, but in case you don't have the time, here is a speedier version.

2 16-ounce cans blackeyed peas, rinsed and drained
1 cup cooked rice
1 tablespoon dehydrated onion flakes
⅛ teaspoon liquid smoke
1 tablespoon imitation bacon bits
hot sauce to taste

Combine all of the ingredients and simmer over medium heat until warmed through.

4 servings
Less than 1 fat gram per serving

Luau Baked Beans

This is a classic example of how vegetables can be used to add bulk to a dish. While you don't have to count calories on a low-fat lifestyle, it is good to add low-fat, low-calorie extenders to dishes whenever possible.

2 green peppers, cut into squares
1 large onion chopped
no-stick cooking spray
1 clove garlic or ⅛ teaspoon garlic powder
2 cans fat-free baked beans
½ cup juice-packed pineapple tidbits, drained
1 8-ounce can sliced water chestnuts, drained

Sauté the green peppers and onions in a skillet that has been coated with no-stick cooking spray. Add the other ingredients. Pour into a casserole dish and bake at 350° for 20 minutes. This is good with ham or grilled chicken.

4 servings
0 fat grams

Red Beans and Rice

This New Orleans favorite has become a favorite around our house too. Traditionally, New Orleans cooks prepared it on wash day, so that the cook could just start the beans and forget them while doing the washing. Then at the end of the long tiring day, dinner was ready without much preparation. My sentiments exactly. I love to come in from work to a slow cooker full of delicious red beans. I know that I can have a nutritious dinner on the table and be out of the kitchen in no time.

1 pound dry kidney beans
6 cups water
2 medium onions, chopped
3 chicken bouillon cubes
¼ teaspoon garlic powder
2 tablespoons chili powder, or to taste
hot sauce to taste

Soak the beans overnight. Pour off the soaking liquid and replace with about 6 cups of fresh water. Place in a slow cooker with the remaining ingredients. Cook for 8-12 hours on low. Serve with rice.

Variation: Can be cooked with 8 ounces 98% fat-free cubed ham.

8 servings
Less than 1 fat gram per serving
if prepared without ham

Versatile Cuban Black Beans

Another bean dish that I serve often. I usually prepare a recipe of the basic beans in the slow cooker. The first day we eat the basic beans on a bed of hot, cooked rice, topped with chopped onions and hot sauce. Later in the week I add a large can of Mexican style tomato sauce and serve it as black bean soup. Anything to cut down on time in the kitchen!

1 pound black beans, picked over and soaked overnight
6 cups water
3 chicken bouillon cubes
1 large onion, chopped
1 green pepper, chopped
1 teaspoon liquid smoke
1 tablespoon cumin, or to taste
1 tablespoon chili powder, or to taste

Carefully pick over the black beans before soaking. After soaking overnight, discard the water and replace with 8 cups fresh water. Add the remaining ingredients. Cook 8-12 hours on low in a slow cooker.

8 servings
Less than 1 fat gram per serving

Broccoli and Potato Casserole
6 medium baking potatoes, peeled and cut into chunks
1 ½-ounce package butter-flavored granules
¼ cup skim milk
1 10-ounce package frozen chopped broccoli, cooked
    and drained
1 teaspoon dehydrated minced onion
4 ounces fat-free Cheddar cheese, shredded
no-stick cooking spray

Boil the potatoes over medium heat until tender. Mash the potatoes. Add the butter-flavored granules, milk, cooked broccoli, dehydrated onion and cheese. Pour into a casserole dish that has been sprayed with no-stick cooking spray. bake at 350° for 15 minutes.

6 servings
0 fat grams per serving

Sesame Broccoli
1 bunch broccoli, trimmed
1 tablespoon soy sauce
1 teaspoon sesame seeds
1 teaspoon sesame oil

Steam the broccoli until tender-crisp. Mix the dressing ingredients together and pour over the broccoli. Serve warm.

4 servings
Less than 1 fat gram per serving

Baked Cabbage
4 cups shredded cabbage
no-stick cooking spray
½ cup skim milk
¼ cup fat-free egg substitute
1 ½-ounce package butter-flavored granules
½ teaspoon poppy seed
salt and pepper to taste

Place the shredded cabbage in a 1 quart casserole that has been sprayed with no-stick cooking spray. Mix the remaining ingredients together and pour over the cabbage. Bake at 350° for 40-45 minutes until the custard is set.

4 servings
0 fat grams per serving

Cabbage and New Potatoes
no-stick cooking spray
2 medium onions, chopped
6 new potatoes, cut into wedges
1½ cups fat-free chicken broth
½ small head of cabbage, chopped

Spray a medium skillet with no-stick cooking spray. Sauté the onion until soft. Add the potatoes and the broth. Cook about 10 minutes over medium heat, covered. Add the cabbage and cook about 10 more minutes.

4 servings
Less than 1 fat gram per serving

Holiday Corn Pudding

A dish from my holiday meal menu from which I have removed the fat. My guests don't seem to miss it.

½ cup fat-free egg substitute
1 cup soft bread crumbs
2 cups skim milk
3 cups cream-style corn
1 ½-ounce package butter-flavored granules
1½ tablespoons sugar or granulated sugar substitute
no-stick cooking spray

Combine the egg substitute, bread crumbs, milk, corn, butter-flavored granules and sugar or sugar substitute. Pour into a casserole dish that has been coated with no-stick cooking spray. Bake for 40 minutes at 350°.

6 servings
0 fat grams per serving

Cheesy Eggplant Casserole

Eggplant has a wonderful meaty quality that makes it a great addition to an all vegetable dinner.

1 medium eggplant, peeled, boiled and mashed
¼ cup fat-free egg substitute
½ of a 10¾ ounce can 99% fat-free cream of mushroom
    soup
½ cup fat-free Cheddar cheese, shredded
½ medium onion, chopped
2 tablespoons catsup
no-stick cooking spray

Combine the eggplant, egg substitute, soup, cheese, onion and catsup. Pour into a casserole dish that has been coated with no-stick cooking spray. Bake at 350° for 35 minutes.

4 servings
1 fat gram per serving

Southern Greens

1 bunch turnip greens, collards or mustard greens
2 chicken bouillon cubes
1 cup water
1 teaspoon light salt

Strip the leaves from the stems and wash thoroughly. Combine all ingredients. Cook in a covered saucepan for 45 minutes or until tender.

4 servings
0 fat grams per serving

Oven Fried Okra

We southerners love our fried okra. This almost fat-free version is not bad. Another alternative is the pre-breaded frozen okra sold in the grocery store. Just read the ingredients label to make sure that oil is not included in the breading.

1¼ cup cornmeal
¼ teaspoon light salt
1½ pound fresh okra, tip and stems removed
no-stick cooking spray

Combine the meal and salt. Slice the okra and coat with the cornmeal mixture. It must be slightly damp for the cornmeal to adhere. Place in a single layer in a shallow pan or iron skillet that has been coated with no-stick cooking spray. Also coat the okra lightly with the spray. Bake at 450° for 30-40 minutes.

4 servings
Less than 1 fat gram per serving

Pepper and Onion Sauté

1 large onion, sliced
2 green peppers, chopped
1 clove garlic, minced or ⅛ teaspoon garlic powder
butter-flavored or olive oil-flavored no-stick cooking
   spray

Sauté the onion, peppers and garlic in a skillet that has been coated with no-stick cooking spray until tender-crisp.

4 servings
0 fat grams per serving

Hash Brown Potato Casserole

It's good to know that many of the frozen hash brown potatoes sold in the grocery store are fat-free. I somehow assumed that they probably had oil as one of the ingredients, since some come ready to cook. The frozen hash brown patties do well sprayed with butter-flavored cooking spray and oven fried, or sautéed in no-stick spray or a teaspoon of oil on the stovetop. This recipe calls for the tiny cubed potatoes that are also sold for use in making hash browns. It's a fat-free version of the old recipe that has been a standby for years.

2 pound bag hash brown potatoes, thawed
1 10¾-ounce can 99% fat-free cream of mushroom soup
1 cup fat-free sour cream
1 cup fat-free Cheddar cheese
1 medium onion, finely minced
light salt and pepper to taste
no-stick cooking spray

Combine all of the ingredients in a casserole dish that has been coated with no-stick cooking spray. Bake at 350° for 45 minutes.

8 servings
Less than 1 fat gram per serving

Irish Potato and Cabbage Casserole

In Ireland this dish is called colcannon. The combination of mashed potatoes and cabbage makes it very filling.

6 medium potatoes, peeled and boiled until tender
¼ cup water
¼ cup skim milk
1 ½-ounce package butter-flavored granules
½ head cabbage, chopped
1 medium onion, chopped
no-stick cooking spray

Mash the potatoes, adding the water, milk and butter-flavored granules. Sauté the cabbage and onion in a skillet that has been coated with no-stick cooking spray. Add the cabbage and onions to the potatoes. Pour the mixture into a casserole that has been sprayed with no-stick cooking spray. Bake at 350° for 15 minutes

6 servings
0 fat grams

Low-fat Potato Patties

2 large potatoes, peeled and grated
1 medium onion, grated
light salt and pepper to taste
1 tablespoon vegetable oil

Combine the potatoes, onion, salt and pepper. Shape into 10 small flat patties. Sauté in the vegetable oil until browned on both sides.

4 servings
4 fat grams per serving

Mashed Potato Casserole

6 medium potatoes, peeled and boiled
3 tablespoons non-fat dry milk powder
½-ounce package butter-flavored granules
½ cup fat-free sour cream
1 medium onion, chopped
4 ounces fat-free Cheddar cheese
light salt and pepper to taste

Mash the potatoes, using as much of the cooking liquid as necessary to achieve the proper consistency. Add the remaining ingredients. Pour into a casserole dish. Bake at 350° for 30 minutes.

4 servings
0 fat grams

Microwave Scalloped Potatoes

4 medium potatoes, peeled and thinly sliced
1 medium onion, thinly sliced
1 tablespoon all-purpose flour
1½ cups skim milk
light salt and pepper to taste

Arrange the potatoes and onion in a 2 quart baking dish. Combine the remaining ingredients and pour over the vegetables. Microwave on high, covered, for 15 minutes. Let stand at least 5 minutes before serving.

4 servings
0 fat grams per serving

Mom's Mashed Potatoes

Some trendy restaurants now serve their mashed potatoes with bits of skin mashed in with the potatoes. You might want to try it for a change of pace. It saves peeling time too! Top each serving with a little fat-free gravy or ultra-low-fat margarine, if desired.

6 medium baking potatoes, peeled or unpeeled, as
    desired, cut into large chunks
1 ½-ounce packet butter-flavored granules
3 tablespoons non-fat dry milk powder
3 tablespoons non-fat sour cream
light salt and pepper to taste

Boil the potatoes until they are tender, then drain. Reserve the cooking liquid. Mash the potatoes until they are free from lumps. Add the butter-flavored granules, the milk powder, sour cream, salt, pepper and enough cooking liquid to achieve the desired consistency. Stir until the ingredients are well blended.

6 servings
0 fat grams per serving

Old Fashioned Creamed Potatoes

2 cups skim milk
3 tablespoons all-purpose flour
1 ½-ounce package butter-flavored granules
4 cups cooked potatoes, peeled and in chunks
light salt and pepper to taste

Add the flour and butter-flavored granules to the milk and cook over medium heat, stirring frequently, until thickened. Add salt and pepper to taste. Add the cooked potatoes and serve.

4 servings
0 fat grams per serving

Oven Fried Potatoes and Onions

4 medium potatoes, peeled and cut into large cubes
1 medium onion, coarsely chopped
1 tablespoon vegetable oil
no-stick cooking spray

Boil the potatoes until half done. This should take about 10 minutes. Drain them well. When cool, place them in a zipper top bag, along with the onion and oil. Shake lightly to distribute the oil. Place the onion and potatoes on a large baking pan with low sides that has been coated with no-stick cooking spray. Bake at 425° for about 25 minutes or until the potatoes are browned. Stir occasionally.

4 servings
4 fat grams per serving

Oven Roasted Potatoes
1 1-ounce envelope dehydrated onion soup mix
5 medium potatoes, unpeeled, cut into chunks
1 onion, chopped
butter-flavor no-stick cooking spray

Preheat the oven to 450°. Combine the soup mix, the potatoes and the onion in a large bowl. Stir gently, so that the vegetables are well coated with the soup mix. Place the vegetables
in a shallow baking dish that has been well coated with butter-
flavor no-stick cooking spray. Spray the vegetables lightly with
the spray. Bake for 40-45 minutes, stirring occasionally until
the vegetables are tender and browned.

4 servings
1 fat gram per serving

Potato Pancakes
1 pound baking potatoes, peeled and grated
3 tablespoons all-purpose flour
1 tablespoon dehydrated onion flakes
light salt and pepper to taste
butter-flavor no-stick cooking spray

Combine the potatoes, flour, onion flakes, salt and pepper.
Form into cakes and sauté in a skillet that has been coated with
butter-flavored no-stick cooking spray.

6 servings
Less than 1 fat gram per serving

Potatoes and Onions in Foil

4 medium baking potatoes
2 tablespoons ultra-low-fat (2 grams per tablespoon)
    margarine
2 medium onions, sliced

Cut each potato crosswise into 4 slices. Spread a bit of the margarine on each slice of potato. Reassemble each potato, placing a slice of onion between each of the potato slices. Wrap each potato in foil. Bake at 375° for 1 hour.

4 servings
Less than 1 fat gram per serving

Skillet Hash Browns

3 medium potatoes, peeled and cut into quarters
1 tablespoon vegetable oil
1 medium onion, minced
½ teaspoon light salt
¼ teaspoon black pepper

Cover the potatoes with water and boil until they are tender. This should take about 10 minutes after the water begins to boil. Drain the potatoes and allow them to cool. (They may be refrigerated at this point for later use.) Cut the potatoes into small cubes and set aside. Heat a large nonstick skillet over medium heat. When the skillet is hot, add 1 tablespoon vegetable oil. Add the onions and sauté until tender. Add the potatoes and continue cooking until the potatoes are browned. Season with the salt and pepper.

4 servings
4 fat grams per serving

Old Fashioned Corn Bread Dressing

I have served this dressing, along with turkey and all the trimmings, for several Thanksgiving and Christmas dinners since I began watching fat grams, and no one has apparently noticed that I took out the entire stick of margarine that I used to add

4 cups corn bread (made from my low-fat recipe), crumbled
2 cups bread crumbs made with reduced-calorie, fat-free bread
3½ cups fat-free chicken broth
1 cup skim milk
½ cup fat-free egg substitute
light salt and pepper to taste
1 tablespoon sage or poultry seasoning
1 large onion, finely chopped
4 stalks celery, finely chopped
no-stick cooking spray

Mix the corn bread and the bread crumbs with the chicken broth. Combine the milk, egg substitute, salt and pepper. Add to the bread mixture. Add the sage or poultry seasoning and the vegetables. Pour into a casserole dish that has been coated with no-stick cooking spray. Bake at 425° for 30 minutes.

6 servings
2 fat grams per serving

Ratatouille

1 medium eggplant, diced
1 medium onion, chopped
2 zucchini, sliced
1 green pepper, chopped
no-stick cooking spray
1 16-ounce can tomatoes, chopped and drained
¼ teaspoon garlic powder
½ teaspoon dried basil
½ teaspoon dried oregano

Sauté the eggplant, onion, zucchini and green pepper in a skillet that has been coated with olive oil no-stick cooking spray. When tender, add the tomatoes and seasonings. Cook for 5 additional minutes.

6 servings
0 fat grams per serving

Spinach and Sour Cream Casserole

3 10-ounce packages frozen chopped spinach, thawed
    and drained
1 10¾-ounce can 99% fat-free cream of mushroom soup
4 ounces fat-free sour cream
½ 1-ounce packet dehydrated onion soup mix.

Combine all ingredients. Pour into a casserole dish and bake at 350° for 20 minutes.

6 servings
Less than 1 fat gram per serving

Holiday Sweet Potatoes

These are the potatoes that I serve, along with my turkey and dressing, at Thanksgiving and Christmas dinner. No one seems to notice that it is any different from my old sweet potato casserole, yet this one has no fat.

6 large sweet potatoes, baked and mashed
sugar substitute to equal 1 cup sugar
½-ounce package butter-flavor granules
½ cup fat-free egg substitute
1 teaspoon vanilla
1 tablespoon grated orange rind
1 tablespoon orange juice
cinnamon and nutmeg to taste
2 cups miniature marshmallows

Combine all of the ingredients, except the marshmallows. Pour into a large baking dish and bake at 350° for 30 minutes. Remove from the oven and top with a single layer of the marshmallows. Briefly run under the broiler until the marshmallows are lightly browned.

6 servings
0 fat grams per serving

Broiled Tomatoes

4 firm ripe tomatoes
butter-flavored no-stick cooking spray
2 tablespoons fat-free Italian salad dressing
2 slices fat-free, reduced-calorie wheat bread, made into
    crumbs
⅛ teaspoon light salt
⅛ teaspoon garlic powder
⅛ teaspoon black pepper

Core the tomatoes and cut in half. Squeeze gently to remove the seeds. Place the tomatoes in a baking dish that has been coated with no-stick cooking spray. Brush the tomatoes with the fat-free Italian dressing. Combine the crumbs and seasoning. Place some of the crumb mixture on each tomato half. Spray each tomato half with the no-stick cooking spray. Bake at 400° for approximately 20 minutes.

8 servings
0 fat grams per serving

Country Style Scalloped Tomatoes

1 medium onion, chopped
½ cup celery, chopped
½ green pepper, chopped
no-stick cooking spray
1 tablespoon all-purpose flour
16-ounce can tomatoes, chopped and undrained
1 tablespoon sugar or granulated sugar substitute
1 teaspoon mustard
3 slices toasted reduced-calorie, fat-free bread, cubed

Sauté the onions, celery and green pepper in a skillet that has been coated with no-stick cooking spray. When the vegetables are wilted, add the flour, undrained tomatoes, sugar or sugar substitute and mustard. Place ½ of the bread cubes in a casserole dish. Top with ½ of the tomato mixture. Repeat the layers. Bake at 350° for 30 minutes.

4 servings
0 fat grams per serving

Oven Fried Green Tomatoes or Yellow Squash

½ cup cornmeal
⅛ teaspoon light salt
¼ cup fat-free egg substitute
1 tablespoon water
3 medium firm green tomatoes or 3 yellow squash,
    sliced into ¼ inch rounds.
no-stick cooking spray

Combine the meal and salt. In a separate bowl, combine the egg substitute and the water. Dip the tomato or squash slices into the egg mixture and then into the cornmeal. Coat a large baking pan with no-stick cooking spray. Place the tomato or squash slices in the pan in a single layer. Coat the slices lightly with the cooking spray. Bake at 450° for 30-40 minutes. Turn the slices halfway through the cooking time.

4 servings
Less than 1 fat gram per serving

Marinated Vegetables

This is the type of dish that is ideal to keep on hand at all times. Not only is it a great side dish with a meal, but it makes a great snack anytime you just have to have something to eat.

1 16-ounce package frozen mixed broccoli, cauliflower
    and carrots
1 medium onion, thinly sliced
½ cup cherry tomatoes, halved
½ cup fat-free Italian dressing

Thaw the frozen vegetables under running water. Drain thoroughly. Combine the drained vegetables with the onion, tomatoes and the Italian dressing. Marinate for several hours.

4 servings
0 fat grams per serving

Microwave Fancy Glazed Vegetables

2 tablespoons brown sugar
2 tablespoons water
½ of ½-ounce package butter-flavored granules
3 carrots, sliced
1 medium onion, cut into wedges
1 cup fresh mushrooms, sliced
2 teaspoons Dijon mustard

Combine the brown sugar, water and the butter-flavored granules in a microwave proof casserole dish. Add all of the vegetables, except the mushrooms. Microwave on high for 2 minutes, covered. Add the mushrooms and cook 8 more minutes. Add the mustard and cook 1 minute longer.

4 servings
0 fat grams

Oven Roasted Vegetable Medley

Many vegetables are good when oven roasted. It is a simple and easy way to cook them.

2 onions, cut into wedges
2 carrots, cut into 1" lengths
2 potatoes, unpeeled, cut into 1" dice
1 eggplant, unpeeled, cut into 1" dice
butter-flavored no-stick cooking spray

Place the vegetables in a single layer in a baking dish that has been coated with no-stick butter-flavored cooking spray. Also spray the vegetables with the spray. Bake at 400° until the vegetables are tender and slightly brown.

6 servings
0 fat grams per serving

Super Simple Casserole

You can use this recipe, to doctor up just about any vegetable or combination of vegetables. Try it with potatoes, eggplant or zucchini.

3 cups cooked vegetable(s)
1 cup fat-free spaghetti sauce
1 tablespoon Parmesan cheese, grated
1 tablespoon dehydrated onion flakes

Combine the vegetable(s), spaghetti sauce and onion flakes. Bake at 350° for 20 minutes. Before serving, sprinkle with the Parmesan.

4 servings
Less than 1 fat gram per serving

GRAINS AND PASTA

These were strictly limited on conventional diets. I love to eat a lot of them because they are so delicious, and especially because they are so filling.

Delicious Barley

Many of us have only eaten barley when we serve canned vegetable or beef soup, which frequently contains this delicious grain. It is important to eat as many whole grains as possible. This is one good way to do it.

1 cup uncooked barley
3 cups water
2 tablespoons instant chicken bouillon granules
1 cup mushrooms, sliced
1 medium onion, chopped
¼ teaspoon garlic powder

Place all of the ingredients in a saucepan and simmer, covered, until done. It will take approximately 40 minutes. Check occasionally to see if additional water is needed.

4 servings
1 fat gram per serving

Basic Bulgur

Bulgur is a wheat product that is very popular in Middle Eastern cooking. It is very versatile and really easy to prepare. It can be purchased in health food stores and larger grocery stores.

1 cup bulgur
3 cups boiling water
1 chicken bouillon cube

Add the bulgur to the boiling water. Simmer for 10 minutes. Remove from the heat and let stand 15 minutes. Drain well.

8 servings
2 fat grams per serving

Bean Burgers and Sausage

With the ultra-low-fat ground beef in the grocery stores and the lower-fat burgers available in restaurants, we can have a hamburger without sabotaging our fat allowance. Granted, some lower-fat burgers can still contain around 10-12 fat grams, but it's worth it sometimes! If you really want the burger without the extra fat, you might try one of the vegetarian burger mixes available in health food stores (some are very good) or you might want to give the following recipe a shot. If you really miss sausage, you might want to try that recipe also.

Bean Burgers

2 cups cooked pinto beans
3 slices fat-free reduced-calorie bread, made into
    crumbs
½ cup egg substitute
½ cup skim milk
2 tablespoons onion, finely minced
¼ teaspoon garlic powder
light salt and pepper to taste
1 tablespoon vegetable oil

Use your hands to "squeeze" everything together, excluding the oil. Shape into patties and sauté in the oil.

Bean Sausage

Follow the directions for bean burgers, omitting the onion and garlic. Add 1 teaspoon sage. Shape into patties and sauté.
17 fat grams per recipe. Divide by # of patties

Delicious Brown Rice

1 cup uncooked brown rice
2½ cups water
1 1-ounce package dehydrated onion soup mix
3 chicken bouillon cubes
1 4-ounce can mushrooms

Combine all ingredients and bring to a boil on the stovetop. Pour into a casserole dish and bake, covered, at 350° for 1 hour or until done.

4 servings
1 fat gram per serving

Deluxe Macaroni and Cheese With Ease

Check out some of the boxed rice and pasta side dish mixes on your grocery store shelves. You may be surprised that many of them have very few fat grams per serving before the milk and butter is added. The brand of macaroni and cheese that I use has 1 fat gram per serving for the dry mix but 13 grams per serving when prepared with milk and butter. The trick is to forget the milk and butter and substitute fat-free goodies.

1 box macaroni and cheese mix (read the label for fat
     content)
½ cup fat-free cottage cheese
½ cup fat-free sour cream

Cook the macaroni according to package directions. When tender, drain all but 1-2 tablespoon water. Add the dry cheese sauce mix and stir. Add the remaining ingredients. Continue cooking on low until the mixture is heated through.

4 servings
1 fat gram per serving

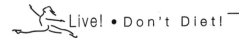

Green Rice

½ cup chopped celery
1 medium onion, chopped
no-stick cooking spray
1 10-ounce package frozen chopped broccoli, cooked
     and drained
1 10¾-ounce can 99% fat-free cream of mushroom soup
½ cup water or fat-free chicken broth
3 cups cooked rice
½ cup fat-free sour cream

Sauté the onion and celery in a saucepan that has been coated with no-stick cooking spray. Add remaining ingredients. Pour into a casserole dish and bake at 350° for 30 minutes.

6 servings
Less than 2 fat grams per serving

Marvelous Millet

Millet is another whole grain that we should eat more often. It is really delicious, and as a whole grain food, is very good for us. You can buy it at health food stores or large grocery stores. It is great served in place of rice or potatoes. A few tablespoons of uncooked millet can also be used as a crunchy topping for casseroles or as a great addition to homemade bread. I seldom make my own bread, but when I do, I always throw in millet to add texture.

1 cup millet
1 teaspoon vegetable oil
2 cups boiling water
2 tablespoons chicken bouillon granules

Sauté the millet in the oil until it is lightly toasted. Add the boiling water and the bouillon granules. Simmer, covered, for 30 minutes.

6 servings
Less than 2 fat grams per serving

Creamy Noodles

1 8-ounce package dry wide noodles, egg free if possible
1 cup fat-free sour cream
1 tablespoon grated Parmesan cheese
1 tablespoon onion, finely minced
1 clove garlic, minced or ⅛ teaspoon garlic powder
1 ½-ounce package butter-flavored granules

Cook noodles according to package directions. Add the remaining ingredients. Serve warm.

4 servings
Less than 2 fat grams per serving

Spanish Rice
2 medium onions, chopped
2 green peppers, chopped
no-stick cooking spray
1 16-ounce can tomatoes, chopped and undrained
1 8-ounce can tomato sauce
1 teaspoon hot sauce, or to taste
1 tablespoon imitation bacon bits, optional
2 cups cooked rice

Sauté the onions and peppers in a skillet that has been coated with no-stick cooking spray. Add the tomatoes, tomato sauce, hot sauce, bacon bits and rice. Pour into a casserole dish and bake at 350° for 30 minutes.

Variation: Add 6 ounces browned ground round, rinsed and patted dry.

4 servings
1 fat gram per serving, if bacon bits are used
3 grams per serving, if ground round is used

THE FAST FOOD LOVER'S LOW-FAT PATH TO HAPPINESS

HOMEMADE LOW-FAT VERSIONS OF FAST FOOD FAVORITES

Most of us have eaten at fast food restaurants all of our lives. We have come to view our fast food favorites as real comfort foods that we just cannot give up. While we can on occasion work fast food treats into our low-fat lifestyles, we may not always want to blow a major portion of our daily fat gram allowance on a high fat fast food favorite. The solution is clear. Make it at home the low-fat way!

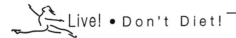

The Almost Fat-free Grilled Cheese Sandwich

The good old grilled cheese sandwich can be made in a way that is almost fat-free. It is tasty, and tons better for you than the old greasy version.

Method One

Heat a griddle on the stovetop. For each sandwich, use 2 slices of 25 calorie per slice, fat-free Cheddar cheese and 2 slices of reduced-calorie, fat-free bread. You may also wish to add 1 ounce of thinly sliced ham or turkey. Spray both sides of the sandwich with butter-flavored no-stick cooking spray. Grill on both sides until golden brown. Add lettuce and tomato.

Method Two

Follow the same directions given for method one, except spread the outside of the bread with approximately 1 teaspoon ultra-low-fat margarine (2 fat grams per tablespoon or less brand).

Less than 1 fat gram per serving, without meat

Amazingly Easy Fat-free Homemade Potato Chips

The key to this recipe is slicing the potatoes super thin. I use an inexpensive plastic slicer that has inserts for thin and thick slicing, as well as chopping. The chips can be served plain or jazzed up with one of the seasoning mixes that you will find in the recipe index.

3 medium size baking potatoes
no-stick cooking spray
light salt or seasoning mix (optional)

Slice the potatoes as thin as possible. Soak the potato slices briefly in cold water. Pat dry. Sprinkle with salt or seasoning, if desired.

Microwave directions: Coat a large, flat plate with no-stick cooking spray. Place a single layer of potato slices on the plate. Microwave on high for 4-6 minutes, or until the chips are crisp and light brown. Rotate the dish halfway through the cooking time. You may also place the potato slices around the inside of a microwave safe plastic colander that has been coated with cooking spray. This allows you to make a few more chips at a time.

Oven Method: Layer the potato slices on a baking sheet that has been coated with cooking spray. Bake at 400° until the chips are light brown.

0 fat grams in the recipe

Baked Corn Dogs
1½ cups self-rising cornmeal mix
½ cup fat-free egg substitute
¾ cup water or more if needed
3 tablespoons applesauce
5 97% fat-free wieners

Combine the cornmeal mix, egg substitute, water and apple-sauce. Space the wieners evenly in a 8" square baking pan. Pour the cornmeal mixture over the wieners. Bake at 425° for 30-40 minutes. Cut apart so that there is a whole wiener in each serving.

5 servings
2 fat grams in each serving

Baked Tortilla Chips
12 corn tortillas
no-stick cooking spray
salt

Lightly spray each tortilla with the no-stick cooking spray. Sprinkle with salt. They may also be sprinkled with chili powder if desired. Cut each tortilla into 6-8 wedges. Place in a single layer on a nonstick baking sheet. Bake in 350° oven for about 10 minutes, or until brown and crisp.

Less than 2 fat grams in 8 chips

Barbecue Sandwiches

Twice a day, every weekday, I must pass one of the best barbecue restaurants in our area. The aroma of the cooking meat that always permeates the air around the restaurant is enough to make you want to forget your best low-fat intentions. One thought alone has saved me. I don't have to be deprived of barbecue. I can just make my own at home the low-fat way with pork tenderloin. At only 4 fat grams per 3- ounce serving, it is a great substitute for other higher fat cuts of pork.

1 pork tenderloin, carefully trimmed of all fat
black pepper, garlic powder and chili powder to taste
1 bottle commercial fat-free barbecue sauce or home-
    made sauce
low-fat or fat-free reduced-calorie hamburger buns

Prepare an outdoor grill for cooking by throwing a handful of water soaked hickory chips on the heat source (charcoal, gas or electric). Rub the tenderloin with a bit of black pepper, garlic powder and chili powder. Cook on the grill, covered if possible, until done. The cooking time will depend on the size and thickness of the tenderloin. It shouldn't take long. Thinly slice the meat, allowing 3 ounces per sandwich. Add a bit of the sauce to a heated bun and pile on the meat. For a restaurant-style touch, you can lightly spray the outside of the bun with no-stick cooking spray and briefly warm the completed sandwich in a skillet or on a griddle until it is slightly toasted.

With fat-free sauce and bun 4 fat grams each.

Broccoli Stuffed Baked Potatoes

Stuffed baked potatoes are becoming a fixture on fast food restaurant menus. The amount of fat in these potatoes is generally quite high. Our homemade version is fat-free.

1 10-ounce package frozen chopped broccoli, cooked
   and drained
1 ½-ounce package butter-flavored granules
4 large baked potatoes
1 recipe fat-free cheese sauce (recipe follows)
4 tablespoons fat-free sour cream

Add the butter-flavored granules to the cooked broccoli. Split the baked potatoes open. Top with ¼ of the broccoli. Add cheese sauce, followed by 1 tablespoon sour cream.

Fat-free cheese sauce:
6 ¾-ounce slices fat-free Cheddar cheese
3 tablespoons skim milk
¼ teaspoon prepared mustard

Tear the cheese slices into strips. Place in a microwave safe measuring cup. Add the milk. Microwave on medium power for less than 1 minute, or until the cheese is melted, stirring frequently. Add the mustard.

4 servings
0 fat grams per serving

Burritos
For each burrito:
2 tablespoons canned fat-free refried beans
1 fat-free flour tortilla, heated to soften
1 tablespoon fat-free sour cream
shredded lettuce
chopped tomato
chopped onion
shredded fat-free Cheddar cheese
bottled taco sauce

Place the refried beans down the center of the tortilla. Add the other ingredients, as desired. Roll the two sides of the tortilla toward the center.

1 serving
0 fat grams per serving

Instant Pizza
Do you ever need a snack or a lunch in a hurry? Try these simple, quick pizzas.

For each pizza:
¼ cup fat-free spaghetti sauce
1 ounce fat-free mozzarella cheese, shredded
1 tablespoon onion, chopped (optional
1 tablespoon green pepper, chopped (optional)
garlic powder and oregano to taste
1 English muffin half, toasted

Layer the topping ingredients on the toasted muffin half. Bake at 350° until the cheese just melts, about 5 minutes.

1 serving
1 fat gram per serving

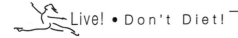

Chicken Nuggets
For each serving:
1 4-ounce chicken breast half, skinned and boned
no-stick cooking spray
¼ cup fine, dry bread crumbs
light salt to taste
pepper
1 teaspoon vegetable oil

Cut the chicken breast into 6 bite size pieces. Coat lightly with no-stick cooking spray. Combine the bread crumbs, salt and pepper. Roll the chicken breast pieces in the crumb mixture. Sauté the chicken pieces in the oil. Serve with Sweet and Tangy Sauce or fat-free barbecue sauce.

Sweet and Tangy Sauce:
2 tablespoons reduced-sugar peach preserves
1 teaspoon prepared mustard
horseradish to taste

Combine all sauce ingredients and blend well.

1 serving
10 fat grams per serving

Deep Dish Pizza

I made up this recipe after seeing endless commercials for a restaurant that served Chicago style pizzas. They would cut into one, exposing layer after layer of cheeses, meats and vegetables. To keep myself from jumping in the car and rushing out to get one, I knew I better come up with a substitute version.

Crust:
1½ cups all-purpose flour
⅓ cup plus 2 tablespoons warm water
1 package dry yeast
½ teaspoon light salt

Combine all ingredients and knead briefly. Cover and set aside in a warm place until doubled. Spread dough on the bottom and up the sides of a 12" deep-dish pizza pan or casserole dish that has been coated with olive oil no-stick cooking spray. Dust with a bit of cornmeal to keep crust from getting soggy, Layer the following ingredients on the crust:

1 cup fat-free cottage cheese mixed with ¼ cup fat-free egg substitute
1 cup mushrooms, sliced
4 ounces fat-free mozzarella cheese
1 cup onion, chopped
1 cup tomatoes, chopped and squeezed dry
oregano, garlic and basil to taste

Bake at 450° for 20-25 minutes.

4 servings
1 fat gram per serving

The Deli Style Sandwich
For each serving:
2 tablespoons fat-free Italian salad dressing
1 hoagie sandwich roll, sliced lengthwise
2 very thin slices precooked ham
2 very thin slices precooked turkey breast
2 ¾-ounce slices fat-free 25-calorie per slice mozzarella
    or Swiss cheese
shredded lettuce
thinly sliced onion rings
thinly sliced green pepper rings
thinly sliced tomato
dill pickle slices
pickled jalapeno pepper rings or mild pickled pepper rings

Sprinkle the salad dressing onto the two cut sides of the bread. Layer the ham, turkey and cheese on the roll. Top with the vegetables to taste.

1 serving
4 fat grams per serving

The Fast Food Burger

For each hamburger:

4 ounces uncooked ultra-lean ground beef or ground top
    round
1½ low-fat or fat-free reduced-calorie sesame seed ham-
    burger buns
no-stick cooking spray
1 tablespoon fat-free Thousand Island dressing
shredded iceberg lettuce
1 teaspoon finely minced mild onion
1 ¾-ounce slice fat-free Cheddar cheese
dill pickle slices

Shape the beef into two very thin patties. Cook until well
done on a ridged griddle that allows any fat in the meat to drip
away. When the meat is almost done, toast the cut side of the
hamburger bun and both sides of the extra half bun on a griddle that has been coated with no-stick cooking spray.

Assemble the hamburger as follows: Place 1½ teaspoons
Thousand Island dressing on the bottom half of the bun. Add
shredded lettuce, cheese, a hamburger patty and a sprinkle of
chopped onion. Top with the extra bun half. Add the rest of the
dressing, shredded lettuce, a hamburger patty, the remaining
onion, several dill pickle slices and the top bun section.

1 serving
7 fat grams per serving if fat-free bun is used

The Fast Food Style Chicken Filet Sandwich

1 low-fat or fat-free reduced-calorie hamburger bun
no-stick cooking spray
1 tablespoon reduced-fat mayonnaise
1 4-ounce pan fried boneless, skinless chicken breast
    half (see recipe index)
lettuce and tomato slices

Lightly toast the cut sides of the bun on a griddle that has been coated with no-stick cooking spray. Spread the bun with the mayonnaise. Layer the chicken breast, lettuce and tomato on the bun.

1 serving
12 fat grams per serving
(Use fat-free mayo and oven fry the chicken breast
without oil to reduce the fat grams to 6 per serving)

The Fast Food Style Grilled Chicken Sandwich

For each sandwich:
1 4-ounce chicken breast half, skinned and boned
½ teaspoon chili powder
½ teaspoon garlic powder
1 tablespoon fat-free Ranch salad dressing
1 low-fat or fat-free soft sandwich roll
lettuce and tomato slices

Sprinkle the chicken with the chili powder and garlic powder. Grill or sauté until completely cooked. Spread the Ranch dressing on each half of the sandwich roll. Layer the chicken, lettuce and tomato on the roll.

1 serving
4 fat grams per serving if fat-free roll is used

Fast Food Style Mini-Burgers

These are sold all over the country as the specialty of several fast food chains. The name of the chain and the burger may differ from area to area, but the wonderful aroma of the cooking beef and onions makes many of us remember these steamy little burgers fondly.

For each hamburger:

1 tablespoon finely minced onion
no-stick cooking spray
1 ounce uncooked ultra-lean ground beef or ground top
 round
1 commercially prepared 2" square ready to serve soft
 roll
mustard
dill pickle slice

Sauté the onion in a skillet that has been coated with no-stick cooking spray. When tender, remove from the skillet. Shape the meat into a very thin 2" square patty. Sauté until well done. Blot the cooked meat with a paper towel to remove any fat on the surface. Return the onion to the skillet. Cut the roll in half crosswise. Place the cut sides on the meat and onion in the skillet and allow the bun to steam briefly. Place the meat and onion on the bun, adding a dollop of mustard and a dill pickle slice. Most people eat 3-4 each. Prepare plenty!

1 serving
4 fat grams per serving

Fast Food Style Roast Beef Sandwich
1 pound cooked eye of round roast, all fat removed
¼ cup beef broth
4 low-fat or fat-free reduced-calorie hamburger buns
no-stick cooking spray
fat-free barbecue sauce
fat-free horseradish sauce (recipe follows)

Thinly slice the roast beef. Pour the beef broth over the beef to keep it moist. Toast the cut sides of the buns on a griddle that has been coated with no-stick cooking spray. Divide the roast beef among the 4 buns. Serve with barbecue sauce or horseradish sauce.

Horseradish sauce:
½ cup fat-free mayonnaise
horseradish to taste

4 sandwiches
8 fat grams per sandwich if a fat-free bun is used

Good Old Sloppy Joes

These are good served as sandwiches or served open faced with mashed potatoes and another vegetable for a full meal.

1 pound ultra-lean ground beef or ground top round,
    browned and rinsed
1 medium onion, minced
1 green pepper, minced
½ cup catsup
½ cup tomato sauce
¼ teaspoon garlic powder
1 tablespoon Worcestershire sauce
toasted fat-free or low-fat hamburger buns

Combine the browned, rinsed ground beef and vegetables in a skillet. Sauté together until the vegetables are tender. Add the catsup, tomato sauce, garlic powder and Worcestershire sauce. Simmer over low heat for 10 minutes. Serve on the toasted hamburger buns.

4 servings
7 fat grams per serving if fat-free buns are used

Heavenly Hot Dogs

In the area where I live, hot dogs are an art form. There are dozens of small hot dog stands around town, each proudly boasting a special secret sauce that takes hours of preparation. I know one man who spends his lunch hour each day eating at a different hot dog stand. When he works his way through all of them, he starts over. People who have moved away have been known to have their favorite hot dog stand ship them a few by air when they can't stand the deprivation any longer. Thanks to the wonderful ultra-low-fat hot dogs now on the market, we can enjoy a good hot dog anytime. I serve them once or twice a week!

Fast and Tasty Hot Dog Sauce:
1 8-ounce can tomato sauce
2 teaspoons chili powder or more, to taste
1 teaspoon cumin
1 teaspoon sugar or granulated sugar substitute
red pepper flakes to taste

Combine the ingredients and simmer over low heat for 5 minutes. Serve on hot dogs, using 97% fat-free wieners and fat-free or low-fat buns. Pile on the onions, kraut and whatever else you like.

1 gram fat per hot dog if fat-free buns are used

Guiltless French Fries

French fries are one of those foods that we would hate to have to give up. While I can't indulge in the real thing, golden, crisp and loaded with fat, I can enjoy a reasonable facsimile to my heart's (and body's) content. They are also much less messy to make! Spice them up with some of the seasoning mixes in the recipe index, if desired.

4 large potatoes, unpeeled or peeled, as desired
butter-flavored no-stick cooking spray
light salt to taste

Preheat the oven to 450°. Slice the potatoes into standard size fries, steak fries or wedges. Coat a 10" x 13" baking pan with the no-stick cooking spray. Place the potatoes in the baking pan in a single layer. Spray the potatoes with the cooking spray. Bake 30 minutes, or until brown, stirring occasionally.

4 serving
Less than 1 fat gram per serving

Lunch in a Pita

2 cups shredded lettuce
½ medium onion, thinly sliced
1 medium tomato, chopped
4 ounces 99% fat-free precooked turkey breast, sliced
    into matchstick size strips
½ cup fat-free Italian salad dressing
2 whole pitas, cut in half to form pockets

Combine the vegetables and the turkey. Add the salad dressing. Fill each pita half with ¼ of the mixture.

4 servings
2 fat grams per serving

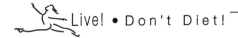

Zippy Mustard Fries
1 tablespoon vegetable oil
1 tablespoon Dijon mustard or prepared mustard
4 medium baking potatoes, cut into strips
no-stick cooking spray

Combine the oil and mustard. Add the potatoes and toss to coat. Place the potatoes in a single layer in 10" x 15" baking pan that has been sprayed with no-stick cooking spray. Bake at 450° for about 30 minutes, stirring every 10 minutes, until brown and crisp.

4 servings
5 fat grams per serving

Nachos
6 ¾-ounce slices fat-free Cheddar cheese
3 tablespoons skim milk
½ teaspoon mustard
baked tortilla chips (See recipe index.)
pickled jalapeno slices

Tear the cheese slices into strips. Combine the cheese strips and milk in a microwave proof measuring cup. Microwave on medium power for less than 1 minute, stirring twice. Add the mustard. Pour the cheese sauce over the tortilla chips. Sprinkle the jalapeno pepper slices over the chips and cheese. Serve immediately.

0 fat grams in cheese sauce
Less than 2 fat grams in 8 chips

The Old Fashioned Hamburger
For each hamburger:
dash Worcestershire sauce (optional)
dash garlic powder (optional)
4 ounces uncooked ultra-lean ground beef or ground
    top round
1 low-fat or fat-free reduced-calorie hamburger bun
mustard to taste
catsup to taste
thinly sliced onion rings
thinly sliced tomato
lettuce
dill pickle slices

Add the garlic powder and Worcestershire sauce to the meat, if desired. Shape the beef into a patty, handling as gently as possible. Either grill outdoors or cook on a ridged stovetop griddle that allows any fat that cooks out of the meat to drip away. Warm the bun, add the cooked hamburger patty, and top with condiments as desired. If you prefer cheeseburgers, add a ¾-ounce slice of fat-free Cheddar cheese.

1 serving
7 fat grams per serving if fat-free buns are used

Oven Fried Onion Rings

French fried onion rings are my weakness. This recipe has kept me from straying when the temptation to indulge in the original version has almost gotten to me.

¾ cup fine, dry bread crumbs
⅛ teaspoon light salt
¼ cup fat-free egg substitute
¼ cup water
2 large onions, sliced into rings
no-stick cooking spray

Combine the bread crumbs and salt. In another bowl, combine the egg substitute and water. Dip the onion rings into this mixture, then in the crumbs. Place on a baking sheet that has been coated with no-stick cooking spray. After the onion rings have been placed on the baking sheet, also coat them with the spray. Bake at 425° for about 15 minutes, or until brown and crisp.

4 servings
Less than 2 fat grams per serving

Philly-Style Cheese Steak Sandwich

For each sandwich:

3 ounces cooked eye of round roast, all fat removed
½ medium onion, thinly sliced
no-stick cooking spray
2 ¾-ounce slices fat-free Cheddar cheese
1 tablespoon skim milk
1 soft low-fat or fat-free sandwich roll

Thinly slice the roast beef and heat until warm. Sauté the onion until limp in a skillet that has been coated with no-stick cooking spray. Meanwhile, tear the cheese slices into small bits. Place them in a measuring cup with 1 tablespoon skim milk. Microwave on medium for 45 seconds, stirring twice. Layer the roast beef on the roll, followed by the onion and the cheese sauce. Wrap in foil and warm in a 350° oven for several minutes.

1 serving
7 fat grams per serving if fat-free buns are used.

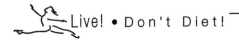

The Reuben-Style Sandwich
For each sandwich:
2 slices low-fat or fat-free rye bread
1 tablespoon fat-free Thousand Island salad dressing
4 deli thin slices 99% fat-free corned beef
1 1-ounce slice fat-free Swiss cheese
¼ cup sauerkraut, drained
no-stick cooking spray

Spread Thousand Island dressing on each slice of bread. Layer the corned beef, cheese and sauerkraut on one slice. Top with the remaining slice. Grill the sandwich on both sides on a griddle that has been coated with no-stick cooking spray.

1 serving
3 fat grams per serving if fat-free buns are used

Snow Cones
Many people remember these treats from trips to fairs or carnivals. They are equally tasty when prepared at home. Most good blenders or food processors will crush ice to a snowy consistency. Just read the directions to make sure your machine is made to crush ice. Use your favorite fruit juice flavors.

For each serving:
1 cup finely crushed ice
1½ tablespoons frozen fruit juice concentrate, thawed

Place the crushed ice in a small paper cup. Drizzle the fruit juice concentrate over the ice. Serve immediately.

1 serving
0 fat grams per serving

Taco Time

I love tacos, but not the fat that you get in take-out tacos or homemade versions that contain regular ground beef. Even store bought taco shells have two grams of fat each. Tacos are kind of like hamburgers. When you dress them up with all the fixings, you can't really tell if there's any meat in them or not.

12 corn tortillas (1 8-ounce package)
1 can fat-free refried beans
shredded lettuce
chopped onions
shredded fat-free cheese
commercial taco sauce

You may use commercially prepared taco shells or save about a fat gram per shell by making your own. Drape corn tortillas over the wires of your oven rack so that they form the traditional taco shape. Heat at 350° until they are crisp. Fill each shell with a heaping spoonful of the heated refried beans, then dress with the toppings you prefer.

Variation: Add 6 ounces browned, well drained ultra-lean ground beef to the refried beans

4 servings
1-2 fat grams per taco without beef

Thin Crust Pizza
Thin crust pizza dough:
1 package dry active yeast
1 cup very warm water (110°-120°)
3½ cups all-purpose flour
1 teaspoon salt
1 tablespoon oil
no-stick cooking spray

Combine the yeast and warm water. In a separate bowl, combine the flour and salt. Add the yeast mixture and the oil to the dry ingredients. Knead the dough until it is smooth and elastic. Let the dough rest, covered, in a warm place for about 1½ hours, or until doubled in bulk. Punch the dough down. Press ½ of the dough into a 12" pizza pan that has been coated with no-stick cooking spray. If the dough resists spreading, let it rest in the pan for ten minutes. Repeat with remaining dough.

Topping:
2 cups fat-free spaghetti sauce or pizza sauce
chopped onion
chopped green pepper
sliced mushrooms
12 ounces fat-free mozzarella cheese, shredded

Divide the sauce and vegetables between the two pizzas. Bake at 425° for 20 minutes. After removing the pizzas from the oven, add half of the shredded cheese to each pizza. Return the pizzas to the oven for 1 minute to melt the cheese.

This recipe makes 2 pizzas.
Each pizza has 9 fat grams.

The Zesty Pizza Burger

For each pizza burger:

4 ounces uncooked ultra-lean ground beef or ground
   top round
1 low-fat or fat-free hamburger bun
2 tablespoons fat-free spaghetti sauce or pizza sauce
1 ¾-ounce slice fat-free mozzarella cheese

Shape the ground beef into a patty, handling as little as possible. Cook on a ridged griddle that allows any fat in the meat to drip away. Place ½ of the sauce on the bottom bun half. Add the cooked hamburger patty. Top with the cheese slice and the remaining sauce. Wrap the burger in foil and place in a 350° oven for 4-5 minutes to melt the cheese and warm the bun.

1 serving
7 fat grams per serving if fat-free buns are used

DESSERTS

I have been known to use a large part of my daily fat gram allowance to indulge in an especially beloved dessert. However, I make desserts an occasional special treat. They are not very filling and often just create a desire for more. When I crave something sweet, a piece of fruit or a cup of diet hot chocolate often is enough to satisfy my sweet tooth.

Almost Fat-free Banana Pudding

2 cups skim milk
2 tablespoons cornstarch
¼ cup sugar
2 teaspoons vanilla flavoring
2 bananas, sliced
12 vanilla wafers

Heat 1½ cups of the milk, stirring constantly. Mix the rest of the milk with the cornstarch and stir until the cornstarch dissolves. Add this mixture to the heated milk. Add the sugar and the vanilla. Cook until thick. When cool, add the sliced bananas. Place 6 of the vanilla wafers in a serving dish. Top with half of the pudding. Repeat the layers. Serve with a dollop of light nondairy whipped topping.

6 servings
2 fat grams per serving

Apple Cobbler

1 20-ounce can light apple pie filling
¼ teaspoon ground cinnamon
1½ cups fat-free baking mix
⅓ cup sugar
¼ cup skim milk

Combine the apple pie filling and the cinnamon. Pour into an 8"x 8" baking dish. Combine the baking mix and sugar. Stir in the skim milk. Drop by spoonfuls on top of the apples. Bake at 350° for 30 minutes.

Variation: Use other light pie fillings, such as peach or blueberry instead of the apple filling.

9 servings
0 fat grams per serving

Frozen Fruit Snacks

Frozen pieces of fruit make a really great and healthy snack. I try to keep some on hand at all times. They are filling and very refreshing, especially when you are hot and tired.

Frozen Bananas

Peel ripe bananas and slice into ¼-inch pieces. Place slices in a single layer on a plate and freeze until firm. Remove the slices from the plate and place in a freezer proof plastic bag, making sure the air is pressed out before sealing. The bananas can also be frozen whole after peeling. This is a good way to use excess bananas before they become too ripe to eat.

Frozen Strawberries

Wash and remove caps from fresh strawberries. Follow the same freezing process used for bananas.

Frozen Seedless Grapes

Select blemish free firm red or green seedless grapes. Follow the same process used for bananas.

Frozen Peach Slices

Peel and slice fresh peaches. Follow the same process used for bananas.

0 fat grams

Belgian Waffle Shortcake
For each serving:
1 Belgian waffle, toasted (Purchase those with 1 fat
    gram per waffle.)
½ cup fat-free vanilla frozen yogurt
1 cup fresh or sugar free frozen strawberries, mashed
    and sweetened with sugar substitute to taste

Place the frozen yogurt on the waffle and top with the strawberries.

Variation: Use fat-free fudge topping instead of strawberries.
1 fat gram per serving

Bread Pudding
6 slices fat-free, reduced-calorie bread, made into
    crumbs
3 cups skim milk
½ cup fat-free egg substitute
½ cup sugar or granulated sugar substitute
¼ teaspoon light salt
¼ teaspoon nutmeg
1 teaspoon vanilla
1 ½-ounce package butter-flavored granules
butter-flavored no-stick cooking spray

Soak the bread in the milk for several minutes. Add the
remaining ingredients. Pour into a baking dish that has been
coated with no-stick cooking spray. Bake at 350° for 30 minutes,
or until a knife inserted in the center comes out clean.
4 servings
0 fat grams per serving

Cinnamon Apples

1 cup water
⅓ cup sugar
½ cup orange juice
1 teaspoon cinnamon
4-5 firm apples, peeled and sliced
1 tablespoon cornstarch dissolved in ¼ cup cold water

Bring the water, sugar, juice and cinnamon to a boil. Simmer 5 minutes. Add the apples. Cover the pot and simmer 20 minutes. Remove the apples. Add the cornstarch mixture to the cooking liquid. Bring to a boil and simmer until thickened. Return the apples to the thickened liquid.

These are good as a dinner side dish, served with ham, or as a pancake topping. You can also serve them warm, topped with ice milk or low-fat frozen yogurt for dessert. For a mock apple cobbler, crumble a cinnamon-sugar graham cracker over a dish of the apples.

4 servings
0 fat grams

Easy Fruit Sorbet

You cannot come up with a less complicated dessert than this one. It is really appealing on a hot summer day. You can make it with any canned fruit that you like. Some possibilities are pineapple, peaches, pears or mixed fruit.

1 16-ounce can of fruit, packed in its own juice, undrained

Puree the fruit and juice in the blender or food processor. Pour into an 8" square pan and freeze until almost firm. Remove from the freezer and break up. Blend again briefly, then return to freezer to finish freezing.

4 servings
0 fat grams

English Trifle

This is a very pretty and light dessert. I usually only serve it when I am having guests. I don't like to keep any leftover trifle around. It is too tempting.

1 large (1.4-ounce) package vanilla sugar-free pudding mix
4 cups skim milk
1 light yellow cake mix
½ cup fat-free egg substitute
1 20-ounce can light cherry pie filling
1 cup light nondairy whipped topping

Prepare the pudding, using the skim milk. Prepare the cake, using the egg substitute. Bake in a 9" x 13" pan. Layer 1" thick slices of the cake in a serving dish. A clear glass dish is preferred. Over the slices of cake place a layer of pudding, followed by a layer of the pie filling. Repeat the layers until all of the cake, pudding, and pie filling have been used. Top with the whipped topping.

Variation: Sliced, fresh strawberries or blueberries can be used instead of the pie filling.

12 servings
5 fat grams per serving

Fat-free Microwave Chocolate Pudding

This can save you when the craving for chocolate gets to you. Knowing that you can fix yourself a big dish of warm chocolate pudding when you get home can get you through watching a fellow diner wade through one of those super fattening chocolate creations that restaurants love to trot out on the dessert cart.

3 tablespoons cornstarch
2¼ cups skim milk
¼ cup sugar
6 packets sugar substitute
¼ cup cocoa powder
2 teaspoons vanilla
⅛ teaspoon salt

Combine the cornstarch and milk. Stir until the cornstarch is dissolved. Add the sugar, the sugar substitute, the cocoa, the vanilla and the salt. Microwave at 100% power for 6 minutes, stirring every 2 minutes

5 servings
Less than 1 fat gram per serving

Fresh Fruit with "Cream" Topping
Topping:
2 cups fat-free cottage cheese
¼ cup skim milk
6 tablespoons sugar or granulated sugar substitute
1 tablespoon vanilla
6 cups fresh fruit

Combine the cottage cheese, milk, sugar or sugar substitute and vanilla in a blender or food processor. Puree until no lumps remain. Serve the topping over the fresh fruit or as a substitute for whipped cream atop any dessert.

6 servings
0 fat grams per serving

Lemon Ice
1 .3-ounce envelope sugar-free lemon gelatin
1 cup boiling water
1½ cups cold water
2 teaspoons liquid sugar substitute
½ cup lemon juice

Sprinkle the gelatin over the boiling water and stir until the gelatin is dissolved. Add the remaining ingredients. Pour in a shallow pan and place in the freezer until the mixture is almost firm. Remove from the freezer and place in a chilled bowl or in the food processor. Beat or process until smooth. Return to the freezer until firm.

4 servings
0 fat grams

Really Lazy Rice Pudding

1 1.4-ounce package sugar-free vanilla pudding
4 cups skim milk
¼ teaspoon nutmeg
2 tablespoons raisins
½ cup cooked rice

Prepare the pudding according to package directions, using skim milk instead of the low-fat milk specified. Add the nutmeg and the raisins, then the rice. Serve chilled.

4 servings
Less than 1 fat gram per serving

Sparkling Fruit Cup

This is a really refreshing variation on the classic fruit in champagne. It is non-alcoholic, and much cheaper to boot.

2 cups apple, peeled and chopped
1 15-ounce can pineapple tidbits (juice packed), drained
2 bananas, sliced
1 cup peaches, peeled and sliced
1 cup seedless grapes
½ cup carbonated lemon-lime beverage

Combine the fruits and chill. At serving time spoon into stemmed dessert glasses. Pour a tablespoon of the carbonated lemon-lime beverage over each portion. Serve immediately.

6 servings
0 fat grams per serving

Sunday Best Baked Apples

¼ cup raisins
3 tablespoons brown sugar
1 teaspoon cinnamon
½ of ½-ounce package butter-flavored granules
4 firm apples, cored
½ cup water

Combine the raisins, sugar, cinnamon and butter-flavored granules. Stuff the apples with the mixture. Pour the water around the apples. Bake at 350° for 45 minutes.

4 servings
0 fat grams per serving

SAUCES AND CONDIMENTS

Sauces and condiments add interest and sparkle to many dishes. Keep a lot of them on hand. I have a large cabinet full of both commercially prepared and homemade condiments of all kinds. I also keep an array of commercially prepared sauces, flavored vinegars and mustards. Many commercial sauces and condiments, with the exception of mayonnaise and mayonnaise-type salad dressing, are either low-fat or fat-free. Just remember to check the label.

Basic White Sauce
¼ cup chicken broth
¼ cup all-purpose flour
¼ cup nonfat dry milk powder
2 cups skim milk
1 ½-ounce package butter-flavored granules

Combine all ingredients. Cook in a saucepan over medium heat, stirring frequently, until thickened.

Uses: Add to vegetables to make creamed vegetables or use to make casserole dishes that call for white sauce.

8 servings
0 fat grams per serving

Easy Cheesy Sauce
This is a quick sauce that is good poured over cooked vegetables, or added to casseroles.

1 10¾-ounce can 99% fat-free cream of mushroom soup
½ soup can water
3 tablespoons fat-free sour cream
4 ¾-ounce slices fat-free Swiss or Cheddar cheese, torn
  into strips

Combine the soup and water in a saucepan. Stir to blend. Place over medium heat. When the soup is hot, add the sour cream and cheese strips. Stir until the cheese is melted.

4 servings
Less than 2 fat grams per serving

Easy Microwave Lemon Sauce

Did you know that gingerbread prepared from a packaged mix is a relatively low-fat treat? This lemon sauce is especially good on gingerbread. It can also serve as a tasty topping for fresh fruit or angel food cake.

½ cup sugar or granulated sugar substitute
1½ tablespoons cornstarch
⅛ teaspoon light salt
1 cup water
2-3 tablespoons lemon juice, to taste

Combine the sugar, cornstarch and salt. Stir in the water. Microwave on high 4-6 minutes, stirring every 2 minutes. Add the lemon juice. Microwave 1 additional minute.

4 servings
0 fat grams

Fat-free Barbecue Sauce

12-ounce can tomato paste
2 cups water
2 tablespoons cider vinegar
2 teaspoons lemon juice
½ medium onion, minced
1 tablespoon Worcestershire sauce
2 tablespoons sugar or granulated sugar substitute
2 teaspoons liquid smoke
1 teaspoon garlic powder
1 tablespoon dry mustard
hot sauce to taste

Combine all ingredients in a saucepan and bring to a boil. Simmer 20 minutes.

0 fat grams in the recipe

Guilt-free Pesto Sauce

A lot of us like pesto, that flavorful pasta sauce that is full of oil and Parmesan cheese. This version is a little more kind to our fat gram allowance.

3 cups fresh spinach
¼ teaspoon garlic powder
1 tablespoon olive oil
¼ cup fat-free sour cream
1 tablespoon Parmesan cheese, grated
1 tablespoon lemon juice

Combine all of the ingredients in a blender or food processor and puree. Serve with pasta.

4 servings
4 fat grams per serving

Fruit Topping

This is a very versatile topping. It can be used on muffins, pancakes or as an ice cream sauce. Try it with peaches or blueberries.

½ teaspoon cornstarch
¼ cup unsweetened apple juice
1 cup berries or sliced fruit
dash of nutmeg
dash of cinnamon

Combine the cornstarch and apple juice. Bring the mixture to a boil, reduce the heat, and simmer until slightly thickened. Add the fruit and spices. Continue to cook until the fruit is heated through.

2 servings
0 fat grams

Great Onion Gravy

This is terrific over mashed potatoes, rice, chicken or vegetables of any kind. On the "rare" occasions that you might treat yourself to a slice or two of eye of round roast, it is especially good with beef.

1 1-ounce package dehydrated onion soup mix
2 cups cold water
2 tablespoons all-purpose flour

Combine the ingredients in a saucepan and bring to a boil, stirring frequently. Continue cooking until thickened.

8 servings
0 fat grams

Salsa Magnifico!

What makes this salsa so magnifico is the fact that it is not only fat free, but almost calorie free also. I keep a jar in the refrigerator all the time. It is not only great served as an accompaniment to Mexican style dishes or with tortilla chips, but also as a quick topping for plain fat-free saltine crackers when you want a simple snack in a hurry.

1 28-ounce can whole tomatoes, undrained
6 ounce can tomato paste
1 medium onion, finely minced
1 green pepper, finely minced
1 4-ounce can diced green chili peppers, undrained
¾ cup cold water
¼ teaspoon garlic powder
¼ teaspoon dried coriander
hot sauce to taste
crushed red pepper flakes to taste

Dice the tomatoes. Mix all ingredients. Keeps indefinitely in the refrigerator.

0 fat grams in the recipe

Tartar Sauce

This classic sauce for seafood is easily prepared using fat-free ingredients. It is also good used as a sandwich spread.

1 cup fat-free mayonnaise
2 tablespoons sweet pickle relish
1 teaspoon dried dill weed
1 tablespoon white wine vinegar

Combine all of the ingredients. Store in the refrigerator and use as needed. Keeps indefinitely.

0 fat grams in the recipe

Apple Relish

4 cups tart, firm green apples, peeled and chopped
1 cup apple cider vinegar
1⅓ cups brown sugar
1 medium onion, chopped
¼ cup raisins
½ teaspoon ground cinnamon
½ teaspoon cloves
1 tablespoon mustard seed

Combine all of the ingredients in a large saucepan. Bring to a boil, then reduce the heat and simmer for 30 minutes, or until the relish is thick. Store in the refrigerator or freeze in pint freezer containers. If preferred, the relish may be canned for future use. Pour the hot relish into hot, sterilized, pint canning jars and process in a boiling water bath for 10 minutes. Makes 2 pints.

0 fat grams in the recipe

Blueberry Chutney

2 12-ounce packages frozen blueberries, unthawed
1 medium onion, chopped
½ cup sugar
1 cup apple cider vinegar
½ cup raisins
1 tablespoon mustard seeds
½ teaspoon ground ginger
½ teaspoon ground cinnamon
¼ teaspoon dried red pepper flakes
light salt to taste

Combine all of the ingredients in a large saucepan. Bring to a boil, then lower the heat and allow to simmer for 45 minutes or until thick. Store in the refrigerator or freeze in pint freezer containers. If preferred, the chutney may be canned for future use. Pour the hot chutney into hot, sterilized, pint canning jars and process in a boiling water bath for 10 minutes. Makes 3 pints.

0 fat grams in the recipe

Chili Sauce From Your Kitchen
4 quarts peeled, chopped fresh tomatoes
2 cups chopped onion
2 cups chopped green peppers
1 cup sugar
3 tablespoons light salt
3 tablespoons mixed pickling spice
1 tablespoon mustard seed
2½ cups cider vinegar

Combine the vegetables, sugar and salt. Tie the spices up in a cheesecloth bag and add them to the mixture. Simmer for about 45 minutes until thick. Add the vinegar and continue cooking briefly. Pour into pint jars, leaving ½-inch headspace. Fasten the lids and process in a boiling water bath for 15 minutes.

Makes approximately 6 pints
0 fat grams

Chunky Mexican Relish
1 16-ounce can chunky Mexican style tomato sauce
½ green pepper, chopped
½ medium onion, finely chopped
1 teaspoon garlic, minced
1 teaspoon cumin
1 teaspoon chili powder

Combine all ingredients. Keeps well in the refrigerator. This is a thick relish and becomes even thicker over time. May be thinned with a bit of water if desired.

0 fat grams

Dried Apricot Chutney
2 6-ounce packages dried apricot halves
2 cloves garlic, minced
1 cup water
1 cup cider vinegar
1 cup sugar
1 teaspoon ground ginger, or to taste

Combine all of the ingredients in a large saucepan. Bring to a boil, then lower the heat and simmer for 20 minutes, or until thick. Store in the refrigerator or freeze in a pint freezer container. If preferred, the chutney may be canned for future use. Pour the hot chutney into a hot, sterilized, pint canning jar and process in a boiling water bath for 10 minutes.

0 fat grams in the recipe

Fresh Cranberry-Orange Relish
This is a delicious relish that is often served at holiday dinners. However, it is a tasty addition to any meal. I like to buy plenty of cranberries and keep them in the freezer, since they freeze beautifully and are sometimes hard to find in stores.

1 pound fresh cranberries, rinsed and drained
1 unpeeled navel orange, quartered
6 tablespoons sugar or granulated sugar substitute

Place the cranberries and orange in a blender or food processor and finely chop. Add the sugar or sugar substitute. Serve chilled.

8 servings
0 fat grams per serving

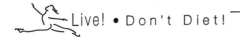

Green Tomato Chutney

2 pounds firm green tomatoes, chopped
4 tart green apples, peeled and chopped
2 medium onions, chopped
½ cup raisins
1 cup sugar
½ teaspoon ground ginger
3 cloves garlic, minced
1¼ cups cider vinegar

Combine all of the ingredients in a large saucepan. Bring to a boil. Reduce the heat and allow to simmer for 30 minutes, or until thick. Store in the refrigerator or freeze in pint freezer containers. If preferred, the chutney may be canned for future use. Pour the chutney into hot sterilized jars and process in a boiling water bath for 10 minutes.

Makes 3 pints
0 fat grams in the recipe.

Microwave Peach Jam

4 cups unsweetened peaches
1 ¾-ounce package powdered pectin
2 tablespoons sugar
½ teaspoon ascorbic acid
1 tablespoon lemon juice

Mash the peaches. Combine with the remaining ingredients in a microwave safe bowl. Microwave, covered, on high for 2 minutes. Stir. Microwave 3-4 more minutes or until the mixture boils for 1 minute. Remove from microwave and let stand 1 minute. Stir again. Will keep in the freezer for up to 1 year or in the refrigerator for several weeks.

0 fat grams per serving

Mixed Fruit Chutney

2 cups peaches, peeled and chopped
2 cups plums, chopped
1 medium onion, chopped
¼ cup brown sugar
2 tablespoons raisins
⅛ teaspoon dry mustard powder
1 tablespoon mustard seed
½ teaspoon ground ginger
½ teaspoon allspice
¼ cup cider vinegar
½ cup orange juice

Combine all ingredients. Simmer about 30 minutes or until thick. Taste and adjust seasoning if needed. Store in the refrigerator or freeze in a pint freezer container. If preferred the chutney may be canned for future use. Pour the chutney into hot sterilized jars and process in a boiling water bath for 10 minutes.

8 servings
0 fat grams per serving

Mom's Chili Sauce

This makes a great relish with bean dishes.

1 15-ounce can diced tomatoes, undrained
chili powder to taste
1 teaspoon vinegar
½ small onion minced
1 teaspoon mustard seed
1 packet sugar substitute

Combine all of the ingredients except the sugar substitute. Simmer until thickened. When cool, add the sugar substitute.

6 servings
0 fat grams

Olden Days Apple Relish

2 dozen ripe tomatoes, peeled and chopped
12 firm cooking apples, peeled and chopped
6 hot peppers
1 dozen medium onions, chopped
4 teaspoons light salt
1½ teaspoons black pepper
2 cups sugar
2 cups vinegar

Combine the ingredients in a large kettle. Boil slowly until thick. Place in pint jars that have been prepared for canning and process in a boiling water bath for 15 minutes.

0 fat grams per serving

Picalilli

1 head green cabbage, chopped
5 firm green tomatoes, chopped
2 medium onions, chopped
2 green peppers, chopped
2 teaspoons pickling salt
1 tablespoon each mustard seed and celery seed
2 cups cider vinegar
1¼ cups sugar

Combine all of the ingredients in a large saucepan. Bring to a boil, then reduce the heat and simmer for 30 minutes, or until the vegetables are tender. Store in the refrigerator or freeze in pint freezer containers. If preferred, the picalilli may be canned for future use. Pour the hot picalilli into hot, sterilized, pint canning jars and process in a boiling water bath for 10 minutes.

Makes 3 pints.
0 fat grams in recipe

Pickled Beets

2 15-ounce cans sliced beets, undrained
2 medium onions, thinly sliced
1 cup apple cider vinegar
1 teaspoon light salt

Combine all of the ingredients. Store in the refrigerator. The beets are ready to eat when the onions turn pink.

4 servings
0 fat grams per serving

Pickled Onion Rings

These are good as an accompaniment to beans. They may also be used on hot dogs or hamburgers, especially in winter when mild onions are often not available.

2 large onions, thinly sliced or chopped if preferred
¼ cup water
½ cup cider vinegar
2 teaspoons light salt
½ cup sugar

Put the onion in a bowl. Combine the water, vinegar, salt and sugar in a saucepan. Heat to boiling. Pour over the onions. Chill 1 hour or longer. The liquid can be reused to make additional onions when needed.

4 servings
0 fat grams per serving

Pickled Pepper Relish

2 cups chopped green pepper
2 cups chopped onion
½ cup sugar or granulated sugar substitute
1 pint cider vinegar
2 teaspoons light salt

Place the peppers and onion in a saucepan. Combine the sugar, or substitute, vinegar and salt. Add them to the pepper and onions in the saucepan. Cook over medium heat until the vegetables are soft and the liquid is slightly thickened. This keeps well in the refrigerator for several months.

8 servings
0 fat grams

MISCELLANEOUS

Crepes

I keep a supply of crepes in my freezer all of the time. They can be used for main courses when filled with meat, side dishes when filled with vegetables, or as dessert when filled with fruit or frozen yogurt.

½ cup all-purpose flour
½ cup fat-free egg substitute
1 cup skim milk
1 tablespoon vegetable oil
no-stick cooking spray

Combine the flour, egg substitute, milk and oil. Let the batter rest in the refrigerator for at least 1 hour before preparing crepes. Spray a crepe pan or a small skillet with no-stick cooking spray. For each crepe, pour ¼ cup batter into the pan. Rotate the pan so that the batter spreads evenly. Bake on one side until the surface is slightly dry and the underside is lightly browned. Turn and cook the other side briefly.

Makes approximately 8 crepes
2 fat grams per crepe

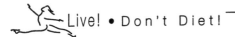

Crisp Salad Croutons

2 plain or onion-flavored bagels, unsliced
butter-flavored no-stick cooking spray
¼ teaspoon garlic powder
¼ teaspoon dried oregano

Cut each bagel into thin coin sized slices. Place each slice on a baking sheet that has been sprayed with no-stick cooking spray. Coat the slices with the spray and sprinkle with the seasonings. Bake at 350° for 15 minutes, or until crisp and toasted, stirring occasionally. Use as a topping for salads.

4 fat grams in the recipe

Delicious "Butter" Spreads

Just because you choose not to blow your fat gram allowance on butter does not mean that you can't enjoy zesty spreads on bread, or added to hot vegetables or grilled chicken.

Easy Garlic Spread

4 garlic cloves, minced, or ½ teaspoon garlic powder
1 tub ultra-light or fat-free margarine

Combine all of the ingredients. Store in the refrigerator and use as needed.

Herb Spread

1 tub ultra-light or fat-free margarine
1 tablespoon chopped chives
1 tablespoon chopped parsley

Combine all ingredients and store in the refrigerator. Use as needed.

Savory Spread

1 tub ultra-light or fat-free margarine
1 tablespoon Worcestershire sauce
2 cloves garlic, minced, or ¼ teaspoon garlic powder

Combine all ingredients. Store in the refrigerator and use as needed.

0 fat grams if fat-free margarine is used
2 fat grams per tablespoon
if ultra-light margarine is used

Fat-free Sour Cream

Before fat-free sour cream became available in grocery stores, it was necessary to make your own. Thank goodness, those days are over! Here's how to make it, in case you want to compare it to the store bought kind.

1 cup fat-free cottage cheese
4 tablespoons skim milk
1 tablespoon lemon juice

Combine all ingredients in a blender. Blend until smooth.

Variations:
Add 1 tablespoon dried or fresh chives to use on baked potatoes.
Add 1 package dehydrated onion soup mix to use as a dip.
Add 2 tablespoons sugar or granulated sugar substitute and 1 teaspoon vanilla to use as a topping for fresh fruit.

4 servings
0 fat grams

Seasoning Mixes For Chips and Fries

Use these mixes to zip up anything. They are great on chips and French fries, but can add extra flavor to a lot of other dishes, from grilled chicken to cooked vegetables. The fat-free sour cream granules and Cheddar cheese-flavored granules can be found in grocery stores in the same section as butter-flavored granules.

Sour cream and onion seasoning mix: Combine 3 tablespoons fat-free sour cream-flavored granules with 3 tablespoons onion powder and ¼ teaspoon light salt.

Spicy seasoning mix: Combine 2 tablespoons chili powder with ½ teaspoon dried cumin powder and ¼ teaspoon light salt.
  Ground red pepper may be added, if desired.

Cheese and garlic seasoning mix: Combine 2 tablespoons fat-free Cheddar-flavored granules with 2 tablespoons garlic powder and ¼ teaspoon light salt.

0 fat grams in each recipe.

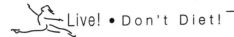

Sweetened Condensed Milk

Commercially prepared sweetened condensed milk is high in fat and calories. This home made version reduces the calories quite a bit and reduces the fat grams to zero. Use in any recipe that calls for sweetened condensed milk, such as lemon ice box pie.

1 cup non-fat dry milk powder
¾ cup granulated sugar
½ cup warm water

Combine all of the ingredients in the top of a double boiler, adding the water a little at the time. If the mixture begins to seem too thin, do not add any more water. Simmer until the milk powder is completely dissolved. Place in the refrigerator. The mixture will continue to thicken as it cools.

0 fat grams in the recipe

Zesty Topping For Casseroles

This recipe is nice to keep on hand to top casseroles. It can also be used as a breading for chicken or fish. Keep a large batch in the freezer in a zipper top freezer bag and use as needed.

12 slices fat-free, reduced-calorie bread
2 teaspoons garlic powder
1 tablespoon grated Parmesan cheese
2 teaspoons dried oregano

Combine all of the ingredients, in a blender or food processor. Blend until the bread is reduced to fine crumbs.

Less than 2 fat grams in the recipe

Index